PUBLIC HEALTH IN THE 21ST CENTURY

SIGNIFICANT HEALTH STATISTICS

SELECT REPORTS FROM FEDERAL AGENCIES

PUBLIC HEALTH IN THE 21ST CENTURY

Additional books in this series can be found on Nova's website
under the Series tab.

Additional e-books in this series can be found on Nova's website
under the e-book tab.

PUBLIC HEALTH IN THE 21ST CENTURY

SIGNIFICANT HEALTH STATISTICS

SELECT REPORTS FROM FEDERAL AGENCIES

CHRISTOPHER BARRETT
EDITOR

nova publishers
New York

Library of Congress Cataloging-in-Publication Data

ISBN: 978-1-63484-563-2

Published by Nova Science Publishers, Inc. † New York

CONTENTS

PREFACE

This book provides significant health statistics through reports from federal agencies. The statistics discussed include updates on previously reported estimates for strategies used by U.S. adults aged 18 and over to reduce their prescription drug costs; regional variation in use of complementary health approached by U.S. adults; health care access and utilization among adults, by race and Hispanic origin; characteristics of hospital stays for super-utilizers by payer; trends in hospital readmissions; hospitalizations for patients aged 85 and over; prevalence of obesity among adults, children and adolescents; sexual activity, contraceptive use, and childbearing of teenagers; serious psychological distress among adults; racial and ethnic disparities in men's use of mental health treatments; and the leading cause of death contributing to decrease in life expectancy gap between black and white populations.

In: Significant Health Statistics
Editor: Christopher Barrett

ISBN: 978-1-63484-563-2

Chapter 1

STRATEGIES USED BY ADULTS TO REDUCE THEIR PRESCRIPTION DRUG COSTS: UNITED STATES, 2013*

Robin A. Cohen, PhD, and Maria A. Villarroel, PhD

KEY FINDINGS

Data from the National Health Interview Survey, 2013

- To save money, almost 8% of U.S. adults (7.8%) did not take their medication as prescribed, 15.1% asked a doctor for a lower-cost medication, 1.6% bought prescription drugs from another country, and 4.2% used alternative therapies.
- Adults aged 18–64 (8.5%) were nearly twice as likely as adults aged 65 and over (4.4%) to have not taken their medication as prescribed to save money.
- Among adults aged 18–64, uninsured adults (14.0%) were more likely than those with Medicaid (10.4%) or private coverage (6.1%) to have not taken their medication as prescribed to save money.

---

* This is an edited, reformatted and augmented version of NCHS Data Brief No. 184, issued by the National Center for Health Statistics, January 2015.

- The poorest adults—those with incomes below 139% of the federal poverty level—were the most likely to not take medication as prescribed to save money.

Approximately one-fifth (18%) of the $263 billion spent on retail prescription drugs in the United States in 2012 was paid out of pocket [1]. Some adults offset the cost of prescription drugs by reducing the dosage and frequency of the recommended pharmacotherapy [2–3]. Other cost-saving strategies include asking providers for less-expensive medications or purchasing medications abroad [4]. This report updates previously reported estimates for strategies used by U.S. adults aged 18 and over to reduce their prescription drug costs [5], using data from the 2013 National Health Interview Survey.

Keywords: medication, expense, National Health Interview Survey

Adults Used Several Strategies to Reduce Prescription Drug Costs

- Almost 8% of U.S. adults aged 18 and over (7.8%) did not take medication as prescribed, to save money; 15.1% asked a doctor for a lower-cost medication, 1.6% bought prescription drugs from another country, and 4.2% used alternative therapies (Figure 1).

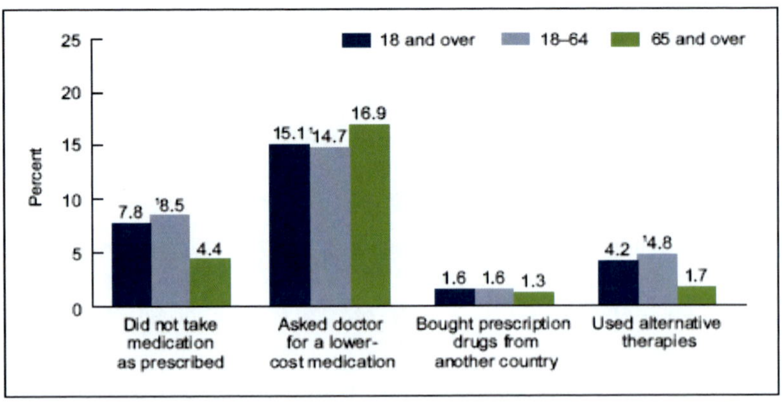

Figure 1. Percentages of adults who used selected strategies to reduce prescription drug costs in the last 12 months, by age group: United States, 2013.

- Adults aged 18–64 (8.5%) were about twice as likely as adults aged 65 and over (4.4%) to have not taken their medication as prescribed to save money.
- Adults aged 65 and over (16.9%) were more likely than adults aged 18–64 (14.7%) to have asked their doctor for a lower-cost medication to save money.
- About 5% of adults aged 18–64 had used alternative therapies to save money on prescription drugs, compared with 1.7% of adults aged 65 and over.
- Less than 2% of adults had bought prescription drugs from another country to save money.

Adults Aged 18–64 Were Almost Twice As Likely As Adults Aged 65 and Over to Have Skipped Doses, to Have Taken Less Medicine, and to Have Delayed Filling a Prescription to Save Money

- Among adults aged 18–64, 5.3% skipped doses and 5.6% took less medication to save money, compared with 2.4% and 2.7%, respectively, of adults aged 65 and over (Figure 2).
- Among adults aged 18–64, 7.2% delayed filling a prescription to save money, compared with 3.4% of adults aged 65 and over.

Among Adults Aged 18–64, Uninsured Persons Were More Likely Than Those with Medicaid or Private Coverage to Have Used Strategies to Save Money on Prescription Drugs

- Adults aged 18–64 who were uninsured were more likely to have asked their doctor for a lower-cost medication (16.5%), to have not taken their medication as prescribed (14.0%), to have used alternative therapies (9.4%), and to have bought prescription drugs from another country (4.2%) to save money, compared with those who had private coverage (14.0%, 6.1%, 3.5%, and 1.0%, respectively) and those who had Medicaid coverage (14.0%, 10.4%, 3.9%, and 0.7%, respectively) (Figure 3).

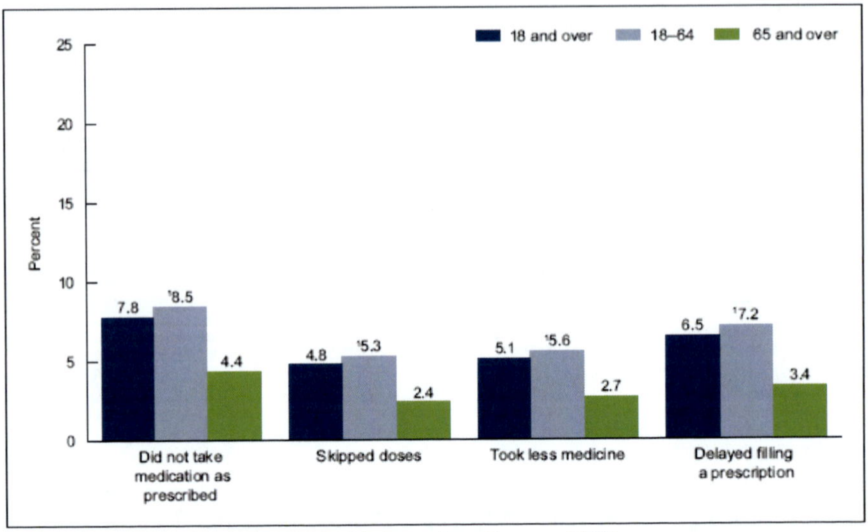

Source: CDC/NCHS, National Health Interview Survey, 2013.

Notes: "Did not take medication as prescribed" is a composite measure that includes adults who "skipped medication doses," "took less medicine," or "delayed filling a prescription." See the Definitions section for further details. A person may use morethan one strategy to reduce prescription drug costs.

[1]Significantly different from adults aged 65 and over ($p < 0.05$).

Figure 2. Percentages of adults who did not take their medication as prescribed in the past 12 months to save money, by strategy and age group: United States, 2013.

- Those who had Medicaid coverage (10.4%) were more likely than those with private coverage (6.1%) to have not taken medication as prescribed to save money.

Among Adults Aged 65 and Over, Strategies Used to Save Money on Prescription Drugs Varied by Insurance Type

- Adults aged 65 and over who had private coverage were less likely to have tried to save money by not taking medication as prescribed (4.0%), compared with those who had both Medicare and Medicaid coverage (6.4%) (Figure 4).

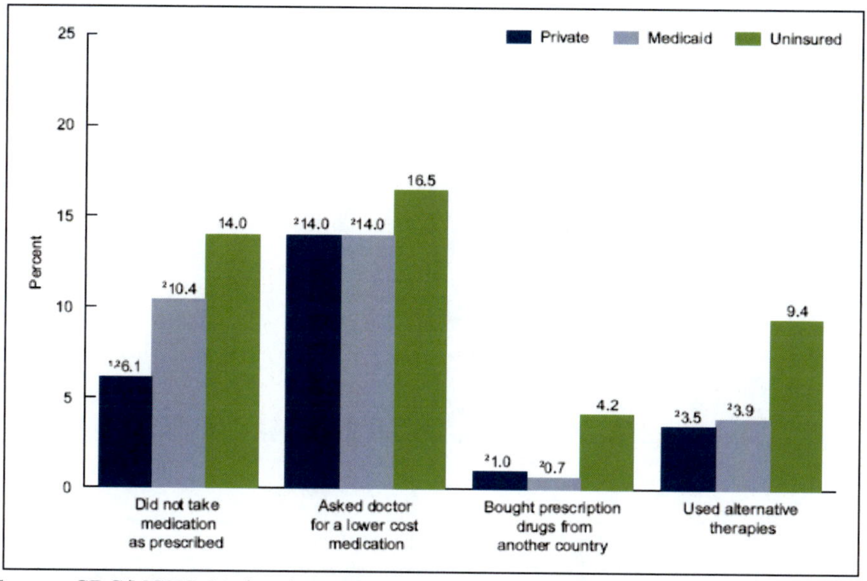

Source: CDC/NCHS, National Health Interview Survey, 2013.

Notes: "Did not take medication as prescribed" is a composite measure that includes adults who "skipped medication doses," "took less medicine," or "delayed filling a prescription." See the Definitions section for further details. A person may use more than one strategy to reduce prescription drug costs.

[1]Significantly different from adults aged 65 and over ($p < 0.05$).2Significantly different from those who were uninsured ($p < 0.05$).

Figure 3. Percentages of adults aged 18–64 who used selected strategies to reduce prescription drug costs in the past 12 months, by health insurance coverage status: United States, 2013.

- Those who had only Medicare coverage (18.1%) or those who had private coverage (18.2%) were more likely to have asked their doctor for a lower-cost medication to save money, compared with those who had both Medicare and Medicaid coverage (12.9%).
- There were no differences by health insurance coverage in the percentage who bought prescription drugs from another country or used alternative therapies to save money.

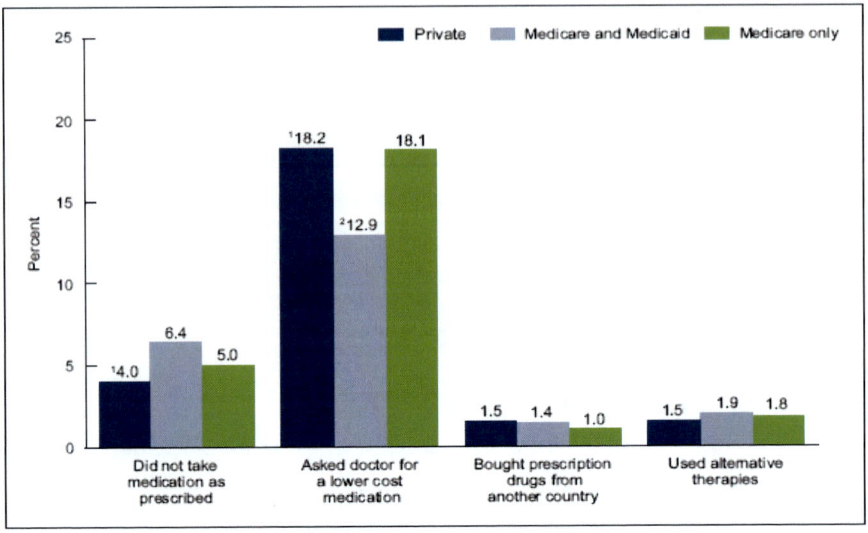

Source: CDC/NCHS, National Health Interview Survey, 2013.

Notes: "Did not take medication as prescribed" is a composite measure that includes adults who "skipped medication doses," "took less medicine," or "delayed filling a prescription." See the Definitions section for further details. A person may use more than one strategy to reduce prescription drug costs.

[1]Significantly different from those with Medicare and Medicaid coverage ($p < 0.05$).2Significantly different from those with Medicare-only coverage ($p < 0.05$).

Figure 4. Percentages of adults aged 65 and over who used selected strategies to reduce prescription drug costs in the past 12 months, by health insurance coverage status: United States, 2013.

The Poorest Adults Were the Most Likely to Not Take Medication as Prescribed to Save Money

- The percentage of adults who did not take medication as prescribed to save money decreased as income increased among all adults aged 18 and over (Figure 5).
- Among adults aged 18–64, the percentage who asked their doctor for a lower-cost medication to save money was highest among those with incomes at or below 250% of the federal poverty level (FPL). The percentages decreased from 17.3% for those with incomes from 139%

through 250% FPL to 12.4% among those with incomes above 400% FPL.

- Among adults aged 65 and over, the percentage who asked their doctor for a lower-cost medication to save money increased from 15.5% among those with incomes below 139% FPL, to 20.9% among those with incomes from 139% through 250% FPL, and 19.7% among those with incomes from above 250% through 400% FPL, and then decreased to 12.7% for those with incomes above 400% FPL.

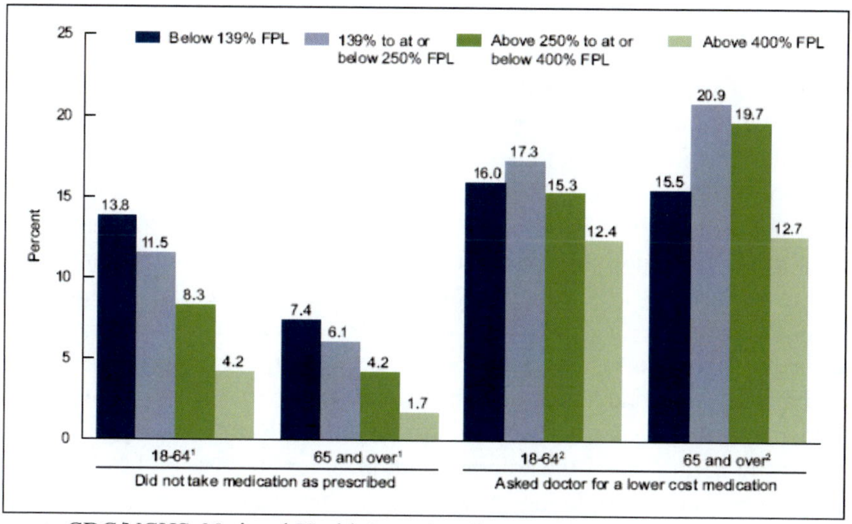

Source: CDC/NCHS, National Health Interview Survey, 2013.

Notes: FPL is federal poverty level. Poverty categories are based on the ratio of the family's income in the previous calendar year to the appropriate poverty threshold (given the family's size and number of children) defined by the U.S. Census Bureau for that year [13]. A person may use more than one strategy to reduce prescription drug costs.

[1]Significant linear trend ($p < 0.05$).

[2]Significant quadratic trend ($p < 0.05$).

Figure 5. Percentages of adults who did not take medication as prescribed and who asked a doctor for a lower cost medication in the past 12 months, by age group and poverty status: United States, 2013.

Summary

Among U.S. adults aged 18–64, strategies for reducing prescription drug costs were more commonly practiced by those who were uninsured than those who had public or private coverage. Lack of health insurance coverage and poverty are recognized risk factors for not taking medication as prescribed due to cost [2]. This cost-saving strategy may result in poorer health status and increased emergency room use and hospitalizations, compared with adults who follow their recommended pharmacotherapy [6–7]. It is unknown whether adverse health outcomes and higher health care costs are also associated with the cost-reduction strategies of alternative therapy use or obtaining prescription drugs from abroad [8–9].

Among adults aged 65 and over, those covered by both Medicare and Medicaid were more likely to have not taken their medication as prescribed to save money, but were less likely to have asked their doctor for a lower-cost prescription, than those who had private insurance coverage. Differences in cost-saving strategies by insurance coverage may be interrelated with socioeconomic and other patient characteristics. Belief that the recommended pharmacotherapy is needed, and an understanding of the recommended treatment, have been found to be lower among older adults who are economically vulnerable, compared with those with higher income [10]. Income was also associated with the use of cost-reduction strategies. Among adults aged 65 and over, those living with incomes at 139%–400% FPL were more likely than adults living in lower or higher income thresholds to have asked their provider for a lower-cost prescription to save money. These patterns in the estimates by insurance status and poverty level are similar to those previously reported using the 2011 NHIS data [5].

Definitions

Strategies for reducing prescription drug costs: Based on the following questions: *The following questions concern the use of prescription medication: During the past 12 months, are any of the following true for you? .[1] You skipped medication doses to save money .[2] You took less medicine to save money ...[3] You delayed filling a prescription to save money ...[4] You asked your doctor for a lower-cost medication to save money .[5] You bought prescription drugs from another country to save money .[6] You used alternative therapies to save money.* In contrast to previous survey years, adults in 2013 were asked questions 1 through 3 only if they reported having been prescribed medication by a doctor or other health care provider during the past 12 months. Adults who were not prescribed medication in the past 12 months are included in the denominator of the estimates pertaining to questions 1 through 3. All adults were asked questions 4 through 6, including those who might not be taking prescription medication.

Did not take medication as prescribed: Based on a positive response to any of the following three questions described previously: *.You skipped medication doses to save money .You took less medicine to save money ... You delayed filling a prescription to save money.*

Health insurance coverage: Respondents were asked about their health insurance coverage at the time of interview. They reported whether they were covered by private insurance, Medicare, Medigap (supplemental Medicare coverage), Medicaid, Children's Health Insurance Program (CHIP), Indian Health Service (IHS), military coverage, a state-sponsored health plan, another government program, or any single-service plans. Adults with both private coverage and some type of public coverage (e.g., Medicaid or Medicare) were classified as having private coverage [11].

Poverty status and percentage of poverty level: Based on reported or imputed family income, family size, and the number of children in the family, and, for families with two or fewer adults, on the age of the adults in the family. Poverty levels are updated annually by the U.S. Census Bureau to reflect changes in the Consumer Price Index. For further information, visit the U.S. Census Bureau website at http://www.census.gov/hhes/www/poverty/poverty.html. Note that NHIS asked respondents about their personal earnings and family income for the previous calendar year (2012). Family income was imputed for 22.7% of persons in 2013 [12].

DATA SOURCE AND METHODS

Data from the 2013 NHIS were used for this analysis. NHIS data are collected continuously throughout the year for the Centers for Disease Control and Prevention's (CDC) National Center for Health Statistics (NCHS) by interviewers from the U.S. Census Bureau. NHIS collects information about the health and health care of the civilian noninstitutionalized population of the United States. Interviews are conducted in respondents' homes, but follow-ups to complete interviews may be conducted over the telephone. The Family component collects information on all family members, and the Sample Adult component collects additional data from one randomly selected adult (the "sample adult"). Questions about strategies to reduce prescription drug cost are from the Sample Adult component. In 2013, information was collected on a total of 34,557 sample adults aged 18 and over. For further information about NHIS, including the questionnaire, see the NHIS website at http://www.cdc.gov/nchs/nhis.htm.

NHIS is designed to yield a nationally representative sample, and this analysis used weights to produce national estimates. Data weighting procedures are described in more detail elsewhere [13]. All estimates shown in this report meet the NCHS standard of reliability (relative standard error less than or equal to 30%). Differences between percentages were evaluated using two-sided significance tests at the 0.05 level.

About the Authors

Robin A. Cohen and Maria A. Villarroel are with CDC's National Center for Health Statistics, Division of Health Interview Statistics.

References

[1] Centers for Medicare & Medicaid Services. National health expenditure data. Available from: http://www.cms.gov/Research-Statistics-Data-and-Systems/Statistics-Trends-and-Reports/NationalHealthExpendData/NationalHealthAccountsHistorical.html.

[2] Briesacher BA, Gurwitz JH, Soumerai SB. Patients at-risk for cost-related medication nonadherence: A review of the literature. *J. Gen. Intern. Med.* 22(6):864–71. 2007.

[3] Piette JD, Rosland AM, Silveira MJ, Hayward R, McHorney CA. Medication cost problems among chronically ill adults in the US: Did the financial crisis make a bad situation even worse? *Patient Prefer Adherence* 5:187–94. 2011.

[4] Nekhlyudov L, Madden J, Graves AJ, Zhang F, Soumerai SB, Ross-Degnan D. Cost-related medication nonadherence and cost-saving strategies used by elderly Medicare cancer survivors. *J. Cancer Surviv.* 5(4):395–404. 2011.

[5] Cohen RA, Kirzinger WK, Gindi RM. Strategies used by adults to reduce their prescription drug costs. NCHS data brief, no 119. Hyattsville, MD: National Center for Health Statistics. 2013.

[6] Heisler M, Choi H, Rosen AB, Vijan S, Kabeto M, Langa KM, Piette JD. Hospitalizations and deaths among adults with cardiovascular disease who underuse medications because of cost: A longitudinal analysis. *Med. Care* 48(2):87–94. 2010.

[7] Jha AK, Aubert RE, Yao J, Teagarden JR, Epstein RS. Greater adherence to diabetes drugs is linked to less hospital use and could save nearly $5 billion annually. *Health Aff.* (Millwood) 31(8):1836–46. 2012.

[8] Herman PM, Poindexter BL, Witt CM, Eisenberg DM. Are complementary therapies and integrative care cost-effective? A systematic review of economic evaluations. *BMJ Open* 2(5):e001046. 2012.

[9] Hubbard WK. Safety of prescription drugs from foreign sources. Statement before the Subcommittee on Human Rights and Wellness, House Committee on Government Reform, June 12, 2003. Available from: http:// www.fda.gov/NewsEvents/Testimony/ucm161056.htm.

[10] Piette JD, Beard A, Rosland AM, McHorney CA. Beliefs that influence cost-related medication non-adherence among the "haves" and "have nots" with chronic diseases. Patient Prefer Adherence 5:389–96. 2011.

[11] Adams PF, Kirzinger WK, Martinez ME. Summary health statistics for the U.S. population: National Health Interview Survey, 2012. National Center for Health Statistics. *Vital Health Stat.* 10(259). 2013.

[12] NCHS. Multiple imputation of family income and personal earnings in the National Health Interview Survey: Methods and examples. Hyattsville, MD: NCHS, Division of Health Interview Statistics. Available from: http:// www.cdc.gov/nchs/nhis/2013imputedincome.htm.

[13] Parsons VL, Moriarity CL, Jonas K, et al. Design and estimation for the National Health Interview Survey, 2006–2015. National Center for Health Statistics. *Vital Health Stat.* 2(165). 2014.

In: Significant Health Statistics
Editor: Christopher Barrett

ISBN: 978-1-63484-563-2

Chapter 2

REGIONAL VARIATION IN USE OF COMPLEMENTARY HEALTH APPROACHES BY US ADULTS*

Jennifer A. Peregoy, MPH, Tainya C. Clarke, PhD, MPH, Lindsey I. Jones, MPH, Barbara J. Stussman, BA, and Richard L. Nahin, PhD, MPH

KEY FINDINGS

Data from the National Health Interview Survey, 2012

- Use of nonvitamin, nonmineral dietary supplements (17.9%) was greater than any other complementary health approach used by U.S. adults in 2012.
- The use of practitioner-based chiropractic or osteopathic manipulation was nearly twice as high in the West North Central region as in the United States overall.

---

* This is an edited, reformatted and augmented version of NCHS Data Brief No. 146, issued by the National Center for Health Statistics, April 2014.

- Use of nonvitamin, nonmineral dietary supplements was highest in the Mountain, Pacific, and West North Central regions.
- Use of yoga with deep breathing or meditation was approximately 40% higher in the Pacific and Mountain regions than in the United States overall.

Complementary health approaches are defined as "a group of diverse medical and health care interventions, practices, products, or disciplines that are not generally considered part of conventional medicine" [1]. They range from practitioner-based approaches, such as chiropractic manipulation and massage therapy, to predominantly self-care approaches, such as nonvitamin, nonmineral dietary supplements, meditation, and yoga. This report presents estimates of the four most commonly used complementary health approaches among adults aged 18 and over in nine geographic regions, using data from the 2012 National Health Interview Survey adult alternative medicine supplement [2].

Keywords: National Health Interview Survey, US regions, chiropractic, dietary supplements

Nonvitamin, Nonmineral Dietary Supplements, Chiropractic or Osteopathic Manipulation, Yoga, and Massage Therapy Were the Most Common Complementary Health Approaches Used in 2012

- The use of nonvitamin, nonmineral dietary supplements (17.9%) was more than twice that of all other complementary health approaches (Figure 1).
- In 2012, chiropractic and osteopathic manipulation was used by 8.5% of U.S. adults, yoga by 8.4%, and massage by 6.8%.
- Other complementary health approaches commonly used by adults in 2012 include meditation (4.1%) and special diets (3.0%).

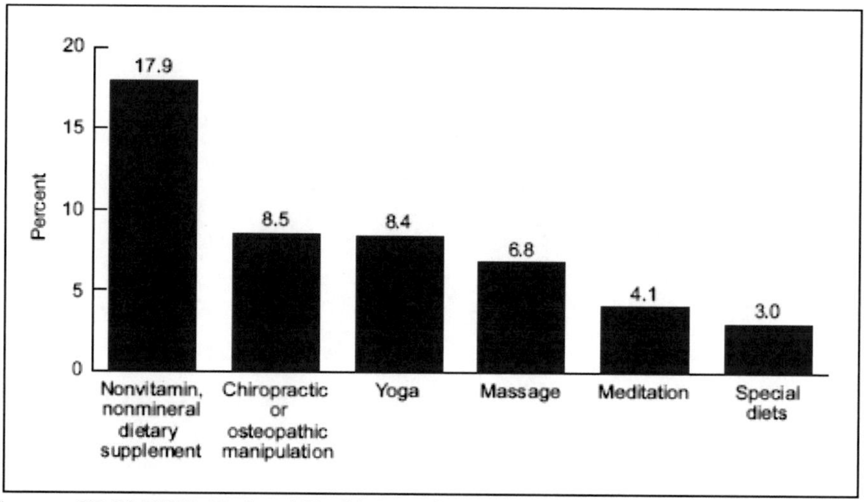

Source: CDC/NCHS, National Health Interview Survey, 2012.
Note: Not all complementary health approaches are presented in this figure.

Figure 1. Percentage of adults who used complementary health approaches in the past 12 months, by type of approach: United States, 2012.

Use of Practitioner-Based Chiropractic or Osteopathic Manipulation Was Twice as High in the West North Central Region as in the United States Overall

- In 2012, 16.4% of adults in the West North Central region, and 11.4% of adults in the Mountain region, used practitioner-based chiropractic or osteopathic manipulation, both of which were higher than the national average (8.5%) (Figure 2).
- Lower use of practitioner-based chiropractic or osteopathic manipulation was found in the East South Central (6.5%), South Atlantic (6.2%), and West South Central (5.9%) regions compared to the national average.
- The Pacific (9.3%) and East North Central (9.5%) regions had similar percentages of practitioner-based chiropractic or osteopathic manipulation use compared to the percentage for the nation as a whole.

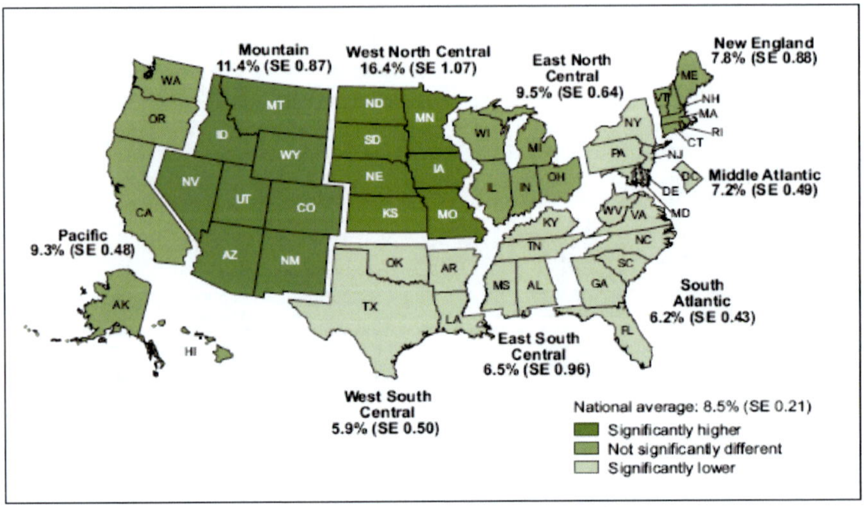

Source: CDC/NCHS, National Health Interview Survey, 2012.
Notes: SE is standard error. Significance is evaluated at the 0.05 level.

Figure 2. Percentage of adults who saw a practitioner for chiropractic or osteopathic manipulation in the past 12 months, by region: United States, 2012.

Adult Use of Nonvitamin, Nonmineral Dietary Supplements Was Highest in the Mountain, Pacific, and West North Central Regions

- The Mountain (28.7%), Pacific (23.3%), and West North Central (23.1%) regions had the highest percentage of adults using nonvitamin, nonmineral dietary supplements (Figure 3).
- The Middle Atlantic (13.6%), West South Central (13.6%), and South Atlantic (13.1%) regions had the lowest percentage of adults using nonvitamin, nonmineral dietary supplements.
- Use of nonvitamin, nonmineral dietary supplements in the East South Central (15.8%) and East North Central (19.5%) regions did not differ from the percentage for the nation as a whole (17.9%).

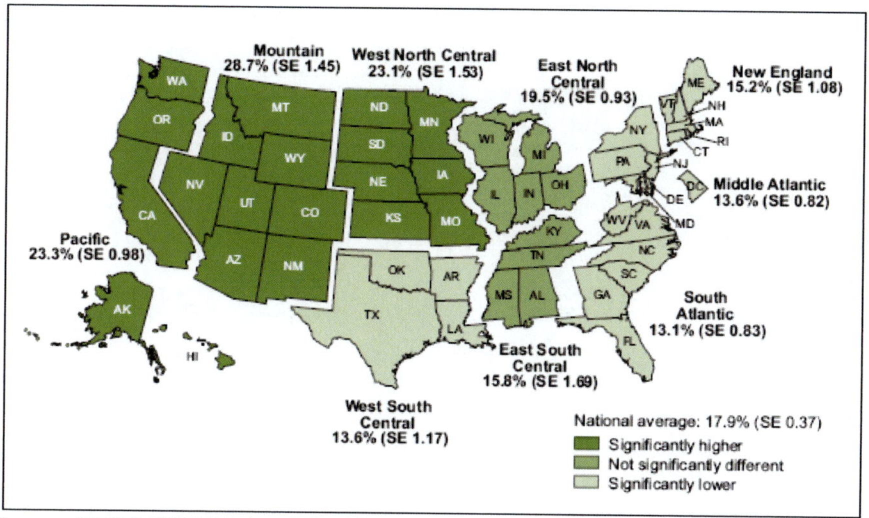

Source: CDC/NCHS, National Health Interview Survey, 2012.
Notes: SE is standard error. Significance is evaluated at the 0.05 level.

Figure 3. Percentage of adults who used nonvitamin, nonmineral dietary supplements in the past 12 months, by region: United States, 2012.

The Use of Yoga with Deep Breathing or Meditation Was Approximately 40% Higher in the Pacific and Mountain Regions Than the National Average

- Yoga with deep breathing or meditation use in the East South Central (5.1%), West South Central (6.0%), South Atlantic (6.8%), and Middle Atlantic (7.1%) regions was lower than the percentage for the nation as a whole (Figure 4).
- When compared to the national average, no significant difference was observed in the percentage of adults who used yoga with deep breathing or meditation in the West North Central (8.7%) and East North Central (8.5%) regions.

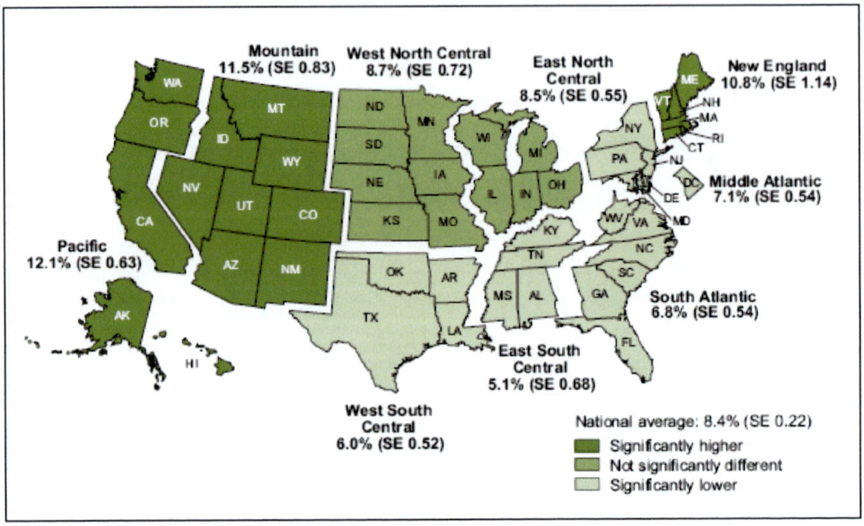

Source: CDC/NCHS, National Health Interview Survey, 2012.
Notes: SE is standard error. Significance is evaluated at the 0.05 level.

Figure 4. Percentage of adults who practiced yoga with deep breathing or meditation in the past 12 months, by region: United States, 2012.

In 2012, Adults Living in the Pacific, Mountain, and West North Central Regions Were Most Likely to Have Used Massage Therapy During the Past 12 Months

- The percentage of adults using massage therapy was higher in the Pacific (9.4%), Mountain (9.4%), and West North Central (8.4%) regions than in the nation as a whole (6.8%) (Figure 5).
- No significant difference was found in the use of massage therapy in the West South Central (5.8%), East North Central (7.0%), and New England (7.3%) regions when compared to the national average.
- Use of massage therapy in the East South Central (2.5%), South Atlantic (5.4%), and Middle Atlantic (5.6%) regions was lower than the national average.

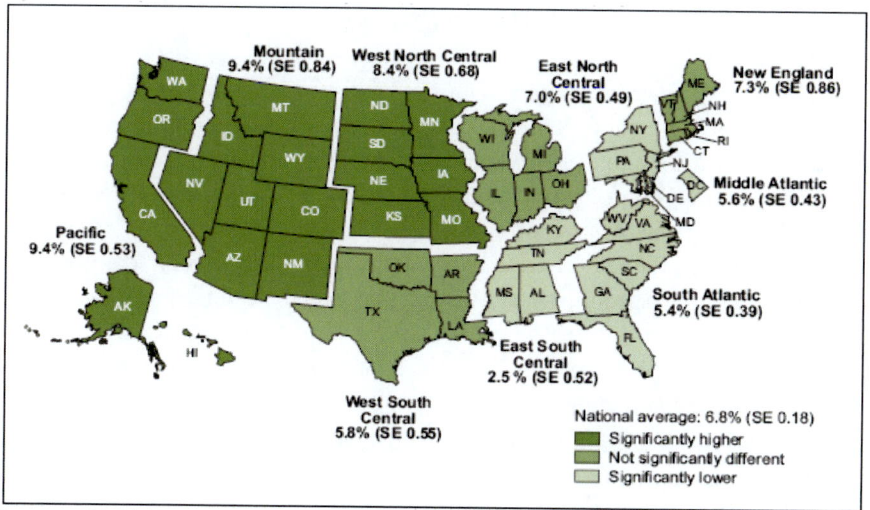

Source: CDC/NCHS, National Health Interview Survey, 2012.
Notes: SE is standard error. Significance is evaluated at the 0.05 level.

Figure 5. Percentage of adults who used massage therapy in the past 12 months, by region: United States, 2012.

SUMMARY

In 2012, nonvitamin, nonmineral dietary supplements (17.9%), practitioner-based chiropractic or osteopathic manipulation (8.5%), yoga with deep breathing or meditation (8.4%), and massage therapy (6.8%) were the most common complementary health approaches used by U.S. adults. Previous research demonstrated that regional differences exist in the use of complementary health approaches among adults in the United States [3, 4], and this report reveals that those regional differences persist across a wide range of complementary health approaches. Environmental and cultural factors unique to towns, regions, and economic factors have long been linked to differences in health behaviors and general health measures in the U.S. population [5]. Similar environmental and cultural factors may be related to the regional differences of complementary health approach uses that are presented in this report.

Definitions

Complementary health approaches: Include acupuncture, Ayurveda, biofeedback, chelation therapy, chiropractic or osteopathic manipulation, craniosacral therapy, energy healing therapy, guided imagery, herbs and other nonvitamin supplements, hypnosis, homeopathy, massage, meditation (mantra, mindfulness, and spiritual), Alexander technique, Feldenkreis, Pilates, Trager psychophysical integration, naturopathy, progressive relaxation, special diets, traditional healers, and yoga (with meditation or deep breathing), tai chi, and qi gong exercises. For more information about specific health approaches, refer to http://nccam.nih.gov/health/atoz.htm.

Chiropractic manipulation: A technique that uses a type of hands-on therapy to adjust problems related to the body's structure, primarily the spine, and its function.

Massage: Manipulation of the body's muscle and connective tissues to enhance the physical functioning of those tissues, and promote relaxation and well-being. It is usually performed by massage therapists.

Meditation: A group of techniques with origins in Eastern religious or spiritual traditions. In meditation, a person learns to focus his or her attention and suspend the stream of thoughts that normally occupy the mind. This practice is believed to result in a state of greater physical relaxation, mental calmness, and psychological balance. In 2012, meditation included mantra meditation (including Transcendental Meditation, relaxation response, and clinically standardized meditation), mindfulness meditation (including vipassana, Zen Buddhist meditation, mindfulness-based stress reduction, and mindfulness-based cognitive therapy), and spiritual meditation (including centering prayer and contemplative meditation).

Nonvitamin, nonmineral dietary supplements: Include herbs and other nonvitamin supplements such as pills, capsules, tablets, or liquids that have been labeled as dietary supplements. This category does not include vitamin or mineral supplements, homeopathic treatments, or drinking herbal or green teas.

Osteopathic manipulation: A full-body system of hands-on techniques to alleviate pain, restore function, and promote health and well-being.

Regions: Categories were slightly modified from the nine U.S. Census Bureau-designated divisions: New England—ME, VT, NH, MA, CT, RI; Middle Atlantic—NY, NJ, PA, DC, DE, MD; East North Central—OH, IL, IN,

MI, WI; West North Central—MN, IA, MO, ND, SD, KS, NE; South Atlantic—WV, VA, NC, SC, GA, FL; East South Central—KY, TN, MS, AL; West South Central—LA, OK, AR, TX; Mountain—NV, NM, AZ, ID, UT, CO, MT, WY; and Pacific—WA, OR, CA, AK, HI.

Special diets: A variety of nutritional approaches ranging from a basic, healthy vegetable-based diet to adopting highly restrictive diets and supplement programs. Some diets are highly restrictive; examples of special diets include Zone, vegan, and Ornish diets.

Yoga: Of Hindu origin, a combination of breathing exercises, meditation, and physical postures used to achieve a state of relaxation and balance of mind, body, and spirit. Survey respondents were classified as having practiced yoga during the past 12 months only if they indicated they had practiced deep-breathing exercises or meditation as part of their yoga exercise.

Data Source and Methods

Data from the 2012 NHIS were used for this analysis. NHIS data are collected continuously throughout the year for the Centers for Disease Control and Prevention's (CDC) National Center for Health Statistics (NCHS) by interviewers from the Census Bureau. NHIS collects information about the health and health care of the civilian noninstitutionalized U.S. population. Interviews are conducted in respondents' homes, but follow-ups to complete interviews may be conducted over the telephone.

In 2012, detailed health information was collected on a total of 34,525 persons aged 18 and over from the Sample Adult component of the survey. For further information about NHIS, including the questionnaire, visit the NHIS website: http://www.cdc.gov/nchs/nhis.htm.

Questions on complementary health approaches were from the 2012 adult alternative medicine (ALT) supplement embedded in the Sample Adult component of the survey. The processes used to develop the 2012 ALT supplement, as well as those fielded in 2002 and 2007, have been previously described [6]. The 2012 NHIS ALT supplement collected information from sample adults on their use of 18 complementary health approaches, which included 10 types of provider-based health therapies. NHIS participants were asked if they used or saw a practitioner for each of these approaches during the past 12 months.

Note that the 2012 questionnaire differed substantially from the 2007 questionnaire. Based on cognitive testing and input from expert panels [6], the definitions of certain modalities were modified to reduce false-positive responses. Data users should take these differences into account when conducting analyses and making comparisons between data from 2012 and previous survey years.

The NHIS ALT data were weighted to produce national and regional estimates. Data weighting procedures are described in more detail elsewhere [7]. Point estimates and estimates of their variances were calculated using SUDAAN software [8] to account for the complex sampling design of NHIS. The Taylor series linearization method was chosen for estimation of standard errors. Differences between percentages were evaluated using two-sided significance tests at the 0.05 level. The estimated standard error of the difference between regional and national estimates accounted for nonindependence of regional and national estimates by incorporating their covariance.

About the Authors

Jennifer A. Peregoy, Tainya C. Clarke, and Lindsey I. Jones are with CDC/NCHS, Division of Health Interview Statistics. Barbara J. Stussman and Richard L. Nahin are with the National Institutes of Health, National Center for Complementary and Alternative Medicine.

References

[1] National Center for Complementary and Alternative Medicine, National Institutes of Health. Exploring the science of complementary and alternative medicine: Third strategic plan, 2011– 2015. NIH publication no 11–7643, D458. 2011.

[2] National Health Interview Survey. Adult alternative medicine supplement. Available from: ftp://ftp.cdc.gov/pub/Health_Statistics/NCHS/Dataset_ Documentation/NHIS/2012/althealt_layout.pdf.

[3] Barnes PM, Powell-Griner E, McFann K, Nahin RL. Complementary and alternative medicine use among adults: United States, 2002.

Advance data from vital and health statistics; no 343. Hyattsville, MD: National Center for Health Statistics. 2004.

[4] Barnes PM, Bloom B, Nahin RL. Complementary and alternative medicine use among adults and children: United States, 2007. National health statistics reports; no 12. Hyattsville, MD: National Center for Health Statistics. 2008.

[5] Hartley D. Rural health disparities, population health, and rural culture. *Am. J. Public Health* 94(10):1675–8. 2004.

[6] Stussman BJ, Bethell CD, Gray C, Nahin RL. Development of the adult and child complementary medicine questionnaires fielded on the National Health Interview Survey. *BMC Complement. Altern. Med.* 13:328. 2013.

[7] Botman SL, Moore TF, Moriarity CL, Parsons VL. Design and estimation for the National Health Interview Survey, 1995–2004. National Center for Health Statistics. *Vital Health Stat.* 2(130). 2000.

[8] RTI International. SUDAAN (Release 11.0.0) [computer software]. 2012.

In: Significant Health Statistics
Editor: Christopher Barrett
ISBN: 978-1-63484-563-2

Chapter 3

HEALTH CARE ACCESS AND UTILIZATION AMONG ADULTS AGED 18–64, BY RACE AND HISPANIC ORIGIN: UNITED STATES, 2013 AND 2014*

Michael E. Martinez, MPH, MHSA, Brian W. Ward, PhD, and Patricia F. Adams

In 2014, U.S. adults could buy a private health insurance plan through the Health Insurance Marketplace or state-based exchanges established as part of the Affordable Care Act. Moreover, some states opted to expand Medicaid coverage to low-income adults. Data from the 2013 and 2014 National Health Interview Survey (NHIS) are used to describe recent changes in health insurance coverage and selected measures of health care access and utilization for adults aged 18–64, by race and Hispanic origin.

Keywords: ethnicity, Affordable Care Act, medical care, National Health Interview Survey

---

* This is an edited, reformatted and augmented version of NCHS Data Brief No. 208, issued by the National Center for Health Statistics, July 2015.

Did the Percentage of Uninsured Adults Change from 2013 to 2014 for Selected Race and Hispanic Origin Subgroups?

- Compared with 2013, the percentage of adults aged 18–64 who were uninsured at the time of interview decreased in 2014 for Hispanic (41.1% to 34.1%), non-Hispanic white (14.5% to 11.5%), non-Hispanic black (24.7% to 17.6%), and non-Hispanic Asian (16.1% to 12.1%) adults (Figure 1).

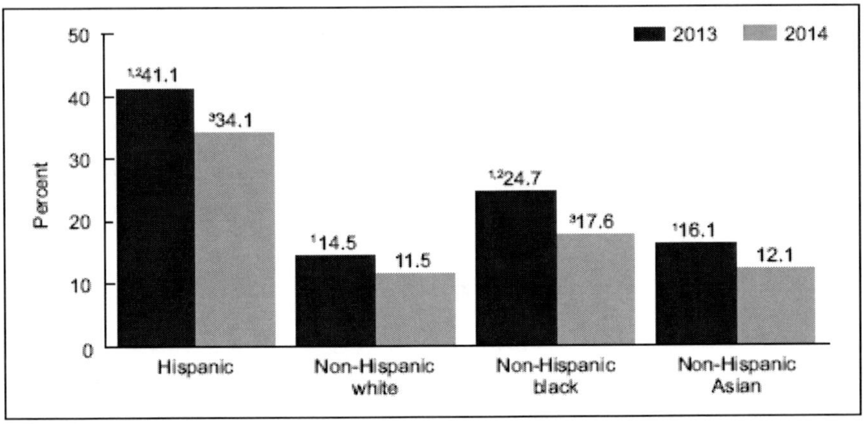

Source: CDC/NCHS, National Health Interview Survey, 2013 and 2014.
[1]Significant difference between 2013 and 2014. 2Significantly different from the other three race and Hispanic origin groups in 2013. 3Significantly different from the other three race and Hispanic origin groups in 2014.

Figure 1. Percentage of adults aged 18–64 who were uninsured, by race and Hispanic origin: United States, 2013 and 2014.

- In 2013 and 2014, Hispanic adults aged 18–64 were the most likely to be uninsured at the time of interview.
- In 2013 and 2014, non-Hispanic white and non-Hispanic Asian adults were the least likely to be uninsured.

DID THE PERCENTAGE OF ADULTS WITH A USUAL PLACE TO GO FOR MEDICAL CARE CHANGE FROM 2013 TO 2014 FOR SELECTED RACE AND HISPANIC ORIGIN SUBGROUPS?

- Compared with 2013, the percentage of adults aged 18–64 who had a usual place to go for medical care increased in 2014 for Hispanic (69.1% to 73.0%) and non-Hispanic white (84.3% to 85.6%) adults (Figure 2).
- The percentage of adults aged 18–64 who had a usual place to go for medical care did not change significantly between 2013 and 2014 for non-Hispanic black and non-Hispanic Asian adults.
- In 2013 and 2014, Hispanic adults aged 18–64 were the least likely to have a usual place to go for medical care.
- In 2013 and 2014, non-Hispanic white adults aged 18–64 were the most likely to have a usual place to go for medical care.

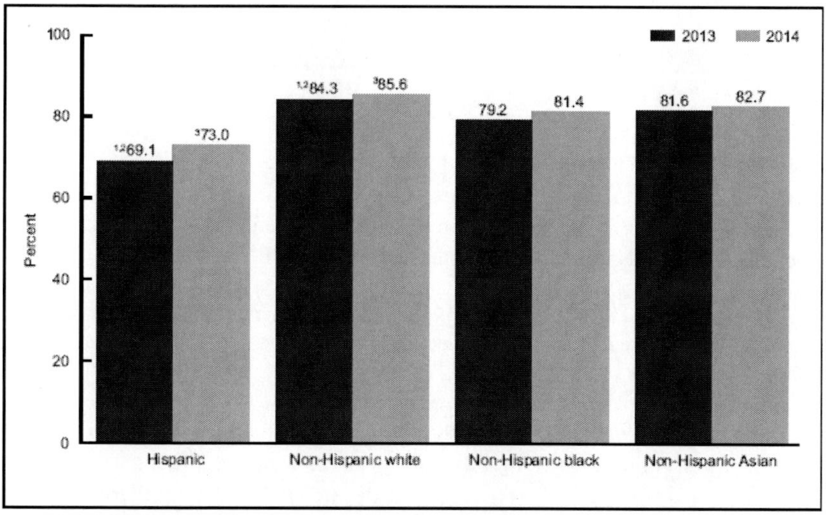

Source: CDC/NCHS, National Health Interview Survey, 2013 and 2014.

Significant difference between 2013 and 2014. 2Significantly different from the other three race and Hispanic origin groups in 2013. 3Significantly different from the other three race and Hispanic origin groups in 2014.

Figure 2. Percentage of adults aged 18–64 with a usual place to go for medical care, by race and Hispanic origin: United States, 2013 and 2014.

Did the Percentage of Adults Who Had Seen or Talked to a Health Care Professional in the Past 12 Months Change from 2013 to 2014 for Selected Race and Hispanic Origin Subgroups?

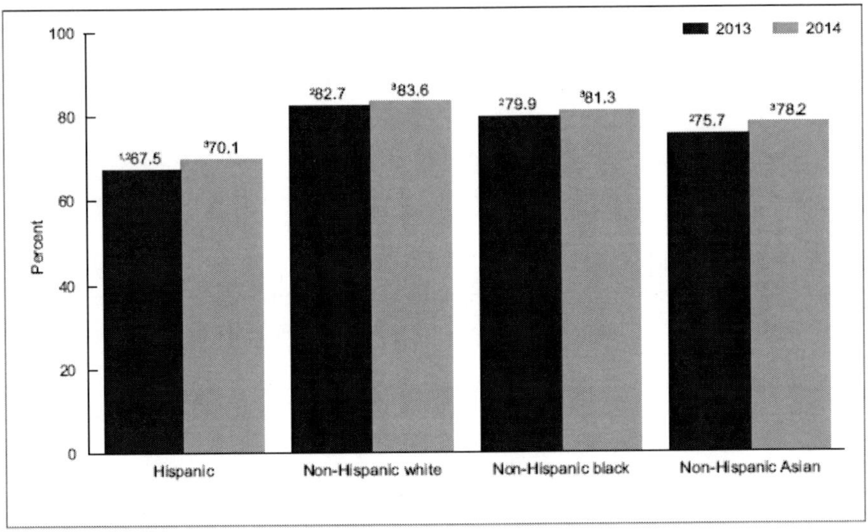

[1]Significant difference between 2013 and 2014.
[2]Significantly different from the other three race and Hispanic origin groups in 2013.
[3]Significantly different from the other three race and Hispanic origin groups in 2014.
Source: CDC/NCHS, National Health Interview Survey, 2013 and 2014.

Figure 3. Percentage of adults aged 18–64 that had seen or talked to a health care professional in the past 12 months, by race and Hispanic origin: United States, 2013 and 2014.

- Compared with 2013, the percentage of adults aged 18–64 who had seen or talked to a health care professional in the past 12 months increased in 2014 for Hispanic adults (67.5% to 70.1%) (Figure 3).
- The percentage of adults aged 18–64 who had seen or talked to a health care professional in the past 12 months did not change significantly between 2013 and 2014 for non-Hispanic white, non-Hispanic black, and non-Hispanic Asian adults.
- In 2013 and 2014, Hispanic adults aged 18–64 were the least likely to have seen or talked to a health care professional in the past 12 months.

- In 2013 and 2014, non-Hispanic white adults aged 18–64 were the most likely to have seen or talked to a health care professional in the past 12 months, followed by non-Hispanic black adults and then non-Hispanic Asian adults.

Did the Percentage of Adults Who Did Not Obtain Needed Medical Care due to Cost Change from 2013 to 2014 for Selected Race and Hispanic Origin Subgroups?

- Compared with 2013, the percentage of adults aged 18–64 who did not obtain needed medical care due to cost at some time during the past 12 months decreased in 2014 for Hispanic (9.9% to 7.6%) and non-Hispanic white (7.7% to 7.0%) adults (Figure 4).
- The percentage of adults aged 18–64 who did not obtain needed medical care due to cost at some time during the past 12 months did not change significantly between 2013 and 2014 for non-Hispanic black and non-Hispanic Asian adults.
- In 2013, Hispanic and non-Hispanic black adults aged 18–64 were the most likely to not obtain needed medical care due to cost at some time during the past 12 months.
- In 2014, non-Hispanic black adults aged 18–64 were the most likely to not obtain needed medical care due to cost at some time during the past 12 months.
- In 2013 and 2014, non-Hispanic Asian adults aged 18–64 were the least likely to not obtain needed medical care due to cost at some time during the past 12 months.

Summary

For all racial and Hispanic origin subgroups examined, there were significant decreases in the percentage uninsured in 2014. Insurance can lead to improvements in health care access and utilization. Indeed, some improvement was observed for some measures of health care access and utilization, especially for Hispanic and non-Hispanic white adults aged 18–64.

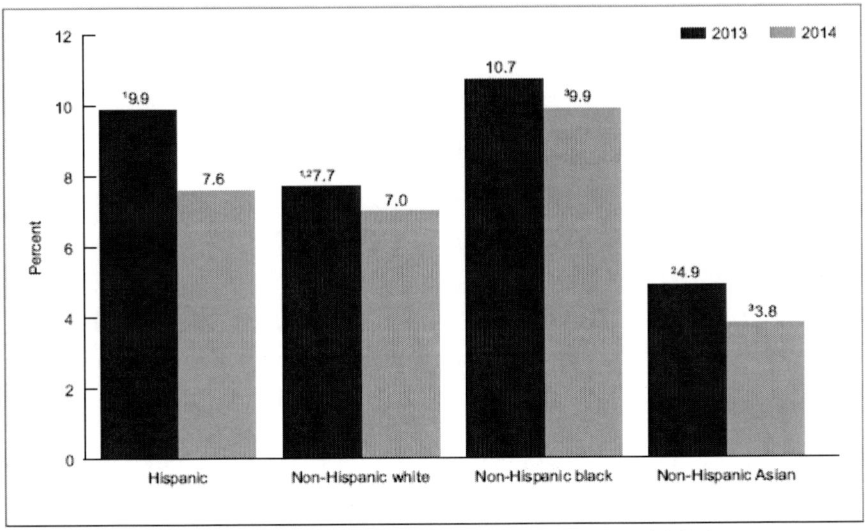

Source: CDC/NCHS, National Health Interview Survey, 2013 and 2014.
[1] Significant difference between 2013 and 2014.
[2] Significantly different from the other three race and Hispanic origin groups in 2013.
3Significantly different from the other three race and Hispanic origin groups in 2014.

Figure 4. Percentage of adults aged 18–64 who did not obtain needed medical care due to cost at some time during the past 12 months, by race and Hispanic origin: United States, 2013 and 2014.

Relative to 2013, Hispanic adults in 2014 were significantly more likely to have a usual place for medical care, were more likely to have seen or talked to a health care professional within the past 12 months, and were less likely to have not obtained needed medical care due to cost at some time during the past 12 months. Relative to 2013, non-Hispanic white adults in 2014 were significantly more likely to have a usual place for medical care and were less likely to have not obtained needed medical care due to cost at some time during the past 12 months. However, compared with 2013, non-Hispanic black and non-Hispanic Asian adults in 2014 did not show any significant improvement across the selected measures beyond the decline in the percentage uninsured.

In 2014, Hispanic adults aged 18–64 were still more likely than non-Hispanic adults to have difficulty accessing and using health care, based on the measures used in this study. Poorer health care access and utilization can lead to poorer health outcomes and higher disease prevalence, which have sometimes been observed for Hispanic adults relative to non-Hispanic white adults [1–3].

DEFINITIONS

Uninsured: A person was categorized as uninsured if he or she did not have any private health insurance, Medicare, Medicaid, Children's Health Insurance Program, state-sponsored or other government-sponsored health plan, or military plan at the time of interview. A person was also categorized as uninsured if he or she had only Indian Health Service coverage or had only a private plan that paid for one type of service, such as accidents or dental care. The analyses excluded persons with unknown health insurance status (about 1% of respondents each year).

Usual place to go for medical care: Based on a question that asked, "Is there a place that you usually go to when you are sick or need advice about your health?" If there was at least one such place, then a follow-up question was asked, "What kind of place [is it/do you go to most often]—a clinic, doctor's office, emergency room, or some other place?" Adults who indicated that the emergency room was their usual place for care were considered not to have a usual place for health care.

Seen or talked to a health care professional in the past 12 months: Based on combined responses of "6 months or less" and "more than 6 months, but not more than 1 year ago" to the survey question, "About how long has it been since you last saw or talked to a doctor or other health care professional about your own health? Include doctors seen while a patient in a hospital."

Did not obtain needed medical care due to cost in the past 12 months: Based on a question that asked, "During the past 12 months, was there any time when [person] needed medical care, but did not get it because [person] couldn't afford it?" Responses exclude dental care.

DATA SOURCE AND METHODS

Data from the 2013 and 2014 NHIS were used for this analysis. NHIS is a multipurpose health survey conducted continuously throughout the year by the Centers for Disease Control and Prevention's (CDC) National Center for

Health Statistics (NCHS). Interviews are conducted in person in respondents' homes, but follow-ups to complete interviews may be conducted over the telephone. Questions about health insurance coverage and not obtaining needed medical care are from the survey's Family Core component, while questions about a usual place to go for medical care and having seen or talked to a health care professional in the past 12 months are from the Sample Adult component. The Family Core component collects information on all family members, and the Sample Adult component collects additional data from one randomly selected adult (the sample adult). For more information about NHIS, including the questionnaire, visit the NHIS website at: *http://www.cdc.gov/nchs/nhis.htm.*

All analyses used weights to produce national estimates. Data weighting procedures are described elsewhere [4]. Point estimates and their estimated variances were calculated using SUDAAN software [5] and the Taylor series linearization method to account for the complex design of NHIS. Two-sided significance tests at the 0.05 level were used to compare estimates. All estimates shown in this report meet the NCHS standard of reliability (relative standard error less than or equal to 30%).

About the Authors

Michael E. Martinez, Brian W. Ward, and Patricia F. Adams are with CDC's National Center for Health Statistics, Division of Health Interview Statistics.

References

[1] Ward BW, Clarke TC, Freeman G, Schiller JS. Early release of selected estimates based on data from the 2014 National Health Interview Survey. National Center for Health Statistics. June 2015. Available from: *http://www.cdc.gov/nchs/nhis/releases.htm.*

[2] Cohen RA, Martinez ME. Health insurance coverage: Early release of estimates from the National Health Interview Survey, 2014. National Center for Health Statistics. June 2015. Available from: *http://www.cdc.gov/nchs/nhis/releases.htm.*

[3] Dominguez K, Penman-Aguilar A, Chang MH, Moonesinghe R, Castellanos T, RodriguezLainz A, Schieber R. Vital signs: Leading causes of death, prevalence of diseases and risk factors, and use of health services among Hispanics in the United States—2009–2013. *MMWR* 64(17):469–478. 2015.

[4] Parsons VL, Moriarity C, Jonas K, et al. Design and estimation for the National Health Interview Survey, 2006–2015. National Center for Health Statistics. Vital Health Stat 2(165). 2014.

[5] RTI International. SUDAAN (Release 11.0.0) [computer software]. 2012.

In: Significant Health Statistics
Editor: Christopher Barrett
ISBN: 978-1-63484-563-2

Chapter 4

CHARACTERISTICS OF HOSPITAL STAYS FOR SUPER-UTILIZERS BY PAYER, 2012*

H. Joanna Jiang, PhD, Audrey J. Weiss, PhD, Marguerite L. Barrett, MS, and Minya Sheng, MS

HIGHLIGHTS

- For this Statistical Brief, super-utilizers were defined as privately insured patients with three or more hospital stays in 2012 or patients covered by Medicare or Medicaid with four or more stays in 2012.
- The average all-cause 30-day readmission rate was four to eight times higher for super-utilizers than for other patients. Among patients aged 1–64 years, super-utilizers accounted for more than half of all 30-day readmissions.
- For all payers, patients with multiple chronic conditions accounted for a greater share of stays among super-utilizers than among other hospitalized patients. For example, among the privately insured, patients with two or more chronic conditions constituted 60.2 percent of all stays for super-utilizers compared with 36.4 percent for other patients.

---

* This is an edited, reformatted and augmented version of Healthcare Cost and Utilization Project (HCUP) Statistical Brief #190, issued by the Agency for Healthcare Research and Quality, May 2015.

- Super-utilizers were more likely to be admitted for medical conditions rather than surgical or other types of conditions. For example, among the privately insured, 65.1 percent of all stays for super-utilizers were admitted for medical conditions compared with 33.3 percent for other patients.
- Common chronic and acute conditions, such as congestive heart failure and septicemia, were among the 10 most common principal diagnoses for hospitalized super-utilizers across all payers.
- Mental health and substance use disorders were among the top 10 principal diagnoses for super-utilizers aged 1 to 64 years regardless of payer.

INTRODUCTION

A large proportion of health care resources in the United States are consumed by a relatively small number of individuals. Approximately one-fourth of U.S. health care expenses are incurred by 1 percent of the U.S. population, and half of expenses are incurred by 5 percent of the population.[1] In contrast, half of the U.S. population incurs only 3 percent of total health care expenses.[2] Those few individuals who consume a large share of health care resources have been dubbed *super-utilizers.*[3] Super-utilizers have become the focus of strategies aimed at reducing their disproportionate use of the health care system by improving the delivery and management of their care.[4,5]

To better understand the characteristics and health care patterns of super-utilizers, the Agency for Healthcare Research and Quality (AHRQ) recently used data from the Healthcare Cost and Utilization Project (HCUP) to examine hospital utilization and costs among Medicaid super-utilizers.[6] The researchers found that, on average, Medicaid super-utilizers had more hospital stays, longer stays, higher hospital costs per stay, and higher hospital readmission rates compared with other Medicaid patients.[7] As payers and providers look to target interventions, it is useful for them to know more about the clinical and demographic profile of super-utilizers.

This HCUP Statistical Brief extends AHRQ's earlier work by exploring characteristics of super-utilizers from other payer groups—Medicare and private insurance—with a comparison to Medicaid super-utilizers. In particular, this Statistical Brief presents data on patient demographics and on resource use and outcomes of hospital stays for super-utilizers compared with stays for other patients by primary expected payer (Medicare, private insurance, and Medicaid). For this report, *super-utilizers* were defined as Medicare or Medicaid patients with four or more hospital admissions or privately insured patients with three or more hospital admissions during 2012 based on a standard cut-off rule applied to the statistical distribution specific to each payer population.[8] The 10 most common principal diagnoses for hospital stays are also identified for these super-utilizers.

Weighted national estimates are produced from the 2012 HCUP Nationwide Readmissions Database (NRD), which includes valid encrypted patient identifiers to allow for tracking across hospital stays and examining readmissions. This analysis includes patients aged 1 to 64 years covered by private insurance, Medicaid (without Medicare listed as a payer), or Medicare, and patients aged 65 years and older covered by Medicare. Differences greater than 20 percent between weighted estimates are noted in the text.

FINDINGS

Patient demographics of hospital stays among super-utilizers by payer, 2012.

Table 1 presents patient demographic characteristics for hospital stays among super-utilizers compared with other patients by payer in 2012.

- For hospital stays covered by Medicaid, on average super-utilizers were older than other patients and women accounted for a smaller share of all hospital stays among super-utilizers than among other patients.

Among hospital stays for patients with Medicaid coverage, on average super-utilizers were older than other patients (40.3 vs. 32.3 years), and the share of hospital stays by women was smaller for super-utilizers than for other patients (50.9 vs. 70.4 percent). In contrast, there were no substantial age or sex differences between hospital stays for super-utilizers and other patients covered by Medicare. Among hospital stays for privately insured patients, the average age was similar for super-utilizers compared with other patients, but women accounted for a smaller share of all hospital stays for super-utilizers than for other patients (53.3 vs. 65.0 percent).

Table 1. Demographic characteristics for hospital stays among super-utilizers[a] by payer, 2012

Characteristic[b]	Medicare aged 65+ years		Medicare aged 1–64 years		Private insurance aged 1–64 years		Medicaid aged 1–64 years	
	Super-utilizers[a]	Other patients	Super-utilizers[a]	Other patients	Super-utilizers[a]	Other patients	Super-utilizers[a]	Other patients
Total number of stays, thousands	1,791	10,075	865	2,384	914	7,192	884	5,297
Mean age, years	77.5	78.0	50.8	52.1	45.3	41.0	40.3	32.3
Female, %	55.2	56.7	49.3	50.8	53.3	65.0	50.9	70.4
Chronic conditions, %								
No chronic condition	1.2	2.4	4.3	7.2	14.2	42.6	10.8	46.5
1 chronic condition	4.8	8.1	10.1	14.2	25.5	20.9	21.4	20.0
2–3 chronic conditions	25.4	35.5	35.8	39.9	37.5	25.7	37.4	21.8
4+ chronic conditions	68.6	53.9	49.7	38.7	22.7	10.7	30.5	11.7

Source: Weighted national estimates from the Agency for Healthcare Research and Quality (AHRQ), Center for Delivery, Organization, and Markets, Healthcare Cost and Utilization Project (HCUP), Nationwide Readmissions Database (NRD), 2012.

[a] Super-utilizers are patients covered by Medicare or Medicaid with four or more hospital stays and privately insured patients with three or more hospital stays in 2012.

[b] Patient demographic characteristics are reported across hospital stays, not across patients. All hospital stays for a patient in 2012 are included in the analysis. The payer-age group classification was identified based on the patient's first hospital stay during the year and applied to all subsequent stays. The statistics presented on patient age, sex, and chronic conditions were identified on the basis of each individual hospital stay.

- Patients with multiple chronic conditions accounted for a greater share of all hospital stays among super-utilizers than among other patients.

For hospital stays covered by private insurance or Medicaid, patients with two or more chronic conditions contributed to a greater share of all hospital stays among super-utilizers than among other patients (private insurance: 60.2 vs. 36.4 percent; Medicaid: 67.9 vs. 33.5 percent). For hospital stays covered by Medicare, only patients with four or more chronic conditions had a higher share of all stays among super-utilizers than among other patients (aged 65+ years: 68.6 vs. 53.9 percent; aged 1–64 years: 49.7 vs. 38.7 percent).

Common principal diagnoses for hospital stays among super-utilizers by payer, 2012.

Table 2 lists the 10 most common principal diagnoses for hospital stays among super-utilizers by payer in 2012. The share of hospital stays attributed to super-utilizers, by payer, also is provided for each of the top 10 principal diagnoses.

Table 2. Top 10 principal diagnoses for hospital stays among super-utilizers[a] by payer, 2012

Principal diagnosis[b]	Rank based on hospital stays by payer				Share of hospital stays attributed to super-utilizers by payer, %			
	Medicare 65+ years	Medicare 1–64 years	Private 1–64 years	Medi-caid 1–64 years	Medi-care 65+ years	Medi-care 1–64 years	Private 1–64 years	Medic-aid 1–64 years
Any principal diagnosis (all stays)	-	-	-	-	15	27	11	14
Congestive heart failure; nonhypertensive	1	6	9	8	28	42	30	36
Septicemia (except in labor)	2	3	5	7	19	28	22	24
Chronic obstructive pulmonary disease and bronchiectasis	3	7		9	24	33		32
Pneumonia (except that caused by tuberculosis or sexually transmitted disease)	4	8	8		17	25	14	
Urinary tract infections	5				18			
Cardiac dysrhythmias	6				13			
Complication of device; implant or graft	7	1	3	10	22	34	28	32
Acute and unspecified renal failure	8				20			
Respiratory failure; insufficiency; arrest (adult)	9	9			24	35		
Complications of surgical procedures or medical care	10	10	2		22	31	26	

Table 2. (Continued)

Principal diagnosis[b]	Rank based on hospital stays by payer				Share of hospital stays attributed to super-utilizers by payer, %			
	Medicare 65+ years	Medicare 1–64 years	Private 1–64 years	Medicaid 1–64 years	Medicare 65+ years	Medicare 1–64 years	Private 1–64 years	Medicaid 1–64 years
Schizophrenia and other psychotic disorders		2		2		31		28
Diabetes mellitus with complications		4	6	3		39	24	32
Maintenance chemotherapy; radiotherapy			1	4			81	74
Mood disorders		5	4	1		26	13	18
Sickle cell anemia				5				57
Alcohol-related disorders				6				33
Secondary malignancies			7				32	
Pancreatic disorders (not diabetes)			10				20	

Source: Weighted national estimates from the Agency for Healthcare Research and Quality (AHRQ), Center for Delivery, Organization, and Markets, Healthcare Cost and Utilization Project (HCUP), Nationwide Readmissions Database (NRD), 2012.

[a] Super-utilizers are patients covered by Medicare or Medicaid with four or more hospital stays and privately insured patients with three or more hospital stays in 2012.

[b] Clinical Classifications Software (CCS) categories based on International Classification of Diseases, Ninth Revision, Clinical Modification (ICD-9-CM) diagnoses. All hospital stays for a patient in 2012 are included in the analysis. Principal diagnoses were identified based on each individual hospital stay.

- Common chronic medical conditions, such as congestive heart failure (CHF), were among the top 10 principal diagnoses for super-utilizers across payers.

CHF was the most common reason for hospitalization among Medicare super-utilizers aged 65 years and older. It also was among the top 10 principal diagnoses for super-utilizers who were younger than 65 years and covered by Medicare, Medicaid, or private insurance. Super-utilizers accounted for around one-third of all CHF hospital stays—28 percent among Medicare patients aged

65+ years, 42 percent among Medicare patients aged 1–64 years, 30 percent among the privately insured, and 36 percent among Medicaid patients.

Chronic obstructive pulmonary disease (COPD) was a top 10 reason for hospitalization for Medicare super-utilizers in both age groups and for Medicaid super-utilizers. Diabetes with complications was a top 10 condition for super-utilizers under age 65 years, regardless of payer. For these two conditions, super-utilizers contributed to about one-third of all hospital stays among patients under age 65 years with Medicare or Medicaid coverage.

- The top 10 conditions for super-utilizers in different payer groups included common acute conditions such as septicemia, pneumonia, and urinary tract infections.

Septicemia was among the top 10 conditions for super-utilizers across all payers—ranked second for Medicare patients aged 65 years and older, ranked third for Medicare patients aged 1–64 years, ranked fifth for privately insured patients, and ranked seventh for Medicaid patients. The share of hospitals stays for this condition attributable to super-utilizers ranged from 19 percent (Medicare aged 65+ years) to 28 percent (Medicare aged 1–64 years).

Pneumonia was a top 10 condition for super-utilizing Medicare patients in both age groups and for privately insured patients. For the younger Medicare age group, super-utilizers accounted for one in four hospitals stays for pneumonia. Urinary tract infection was another top 10 condition for Medicare super-utilizers but only among those 65 years and older.

- Mood disorders were among the top 10 principal diagnoses for super-utilizers aged 1–64 years who were covered by Medicare, Medicaid, or private insurance.

Mood disorders were among the top 10 principal diagnoses for patients aged 1–64 years across all payers, but not for Medicare patients aged 65 years and older. Specifically, mood disorders was the most common reason for hospitalization among Medicaid super-utilizers; it was also a top 10 condition for Medicare and privately insured super-utilizers aged 1–64 years.

Other mental health and substance use disorders also were among the most common diagnoses for super-utilizers for some payers. Schizophrenia was the second most common condition for super-utilizers aged 1–64 years who were covered by Medicare or Medicaid. The share of hospital stays for this condition attributable to these super-utilizers was 31 percent among Medicare patients and 28 percent among Medicaid patients.

Alcohol-related disorders was a top 10 condition for Medicaid super-utilizers, who accounted for one-third of all hospital stays for this condition.

- Cancer-related hospital stays were common among super-utilizing privately insured and Medicaid patients.

Chemotherapy/radiotherapy was the most common reason for hospitalization for privately insured super-utilizers and the fourth most common reason for Medicaid super-utilizers. Super-utilizers constituted the vast majority of all hospitalizations for chemotherapy/radiotherapy: 81 percent of stays among privately insured patients and 74 percent of stays among Medicaid patients. Secondary malignancies also was a top 10 condition for super-utilizers with private insurance.

- Complication of device and complications of surgical procedures or medical care were among the top 10 conditions for super-utilizers in various payer groups.

Complication of medical device was a top 10 reason for hospitalization among super-utilizers across all payers and ranked first among Medicare super-utilizers aged 1–64 years. For this condition, the share of hospitals stays attributable to super-utilizers ranged from about one in three (Medicare aged 1–64 years) to about one in five (Medicare aged 65+ years).

Complications of surgical procedures or medical care was another top 10 condition for super-utilizing Medicare patients in both age groups and for super-utilizing privately insured patients. Among Medicare patients, super-utilizers contributed to 31 percent of all stays for this condition among those aged 1–64 years and 22 percent among those aged 65+ years.

Table 3 presents information on hospital stays, hospital length of stay, hospital costs, readmissions, and types of hospital stays among super-utilizers compared with other patients by payer in 2012.

- An average super-utilizer had approximately four times as many hospital stays per year as did other patients.

Super-utilizers were admitted to the hospital four to six times on average in 1 year. Across all payers, an average super-utilizer had approximately four times as many hospital stays as did other patients. In contrast, among other patients, the average number of stays ranged from 1.1 (private insurance) to 1.5 (Medicare aged 1–64 years).

Table 3. Resource use and outcomes of hospital stays for super-utilizers[a] by payer, 2012

Resource use, outcome	Medicare aged 65+ years		Medicare aged 1–64 years		Private insurance aged 1–64 years		Medicaid aged 1–64 years	
	Super-utilizersa	Other patients	Super-utilizers[a]	Other patients	Super-utilizers[a]	Other patients	Super-utilizers[a]	Other patients
Mean number of stays per year	4.9	1.4	5.7	1.5	4.0	1.1	5.9	1.3
Mean length of stay, days	6.3	5.3	6.3	5.6	5.9	3.6	6.1	4.5
Mean hospital costs, $	12,900	13,000	12,500	13,000	14,600	10,200	11,800	9,000
Aggregate hospital costs, $ (billions)	22.7	128.6	10.7	30.7	12.9	70.5	10.4	47.6
Rate of 30-day all-cause readmissions, %	45.7	11.4	48.1	12.0	44.5	5.1	52.4	8.8
Type of hospital stay, %								
Medical stay	80.1	64.7	70.8	57.8	65.1	33.3	67.0	35.3
Surgical stay	14.3	26.7	13.1	24.4	21.8	30.0	9.0	12.5
Mental health stay	2.3	2.2	13.6	12.2	7.7	5.7	19.3	11.6
Injury stay	3.3	6.5	2.2	4.1	1.8	4.7	2.0	3.8
Maternal/neonatal stay	0.0	0.0	0.3	1.4	3.6	26.3	2.7	36.8

Source: Weighted national estimates from the Agency for Healthcare Research and Quality (AHRQ), Center for Delivery, Organization, and Markets, Healthcare Cost and Utilization Project (HCUP), Nationwide Readmissions Database (NRD), 2012.

[a] Super-utilizers are Medicare or Medicaid patients with four or more hospital stays and privately insured patients with three or more hospital stays in 2012.

- Super-utilizers had an average all-cause 30-day readmission rate that was four to eight times higher than the readmission rate for other patients.

The rate of all-cause 30-day readmissions was much higher among super-utilizers than among other patients, ranging from four times higher (among Medicare patients) to almost nine times higher (among the privately insured).

Across payers, the 30-day readmission rate among super-utilizers was in the 45–52 percent range compared with 5–12 percent among other patients.

- Compared with other patients, Medicaid and privately insured super-utilizers had longer hospital stays and higher average hospital costs.

Compared with other Medicaid patients, Medicaid super-utilizers had stays that were approximately 30 percent longer (6.1 vs. 4.5 days) and average hospital costs that were 30 percent higher ($11,800 vs. $9,000). Similarly, compared with other privately insured patients, privately insured super-utilizers had stays that were approximately 62 percent longer (5.9 vs. 3.6 days) and average hospital costs that were 43 percent higher ($14,600 vs. $10,200). There were no substantial differences in average length of stay or average hospital costs between Medicare super-utilizers and other Medicare patients.

Overall, super-utilizers accounted for between approximately 15 and 26 percent of aggregate hospital costs: 15.0 percent for Medicare patients aged 65+ years, 25.9 percent for Medicare patients aged 1–64 years, 15.4 percent for the privately insured, and 17.9 percent for Medicaid patients.

- Medical stays constituted a greater share of hospitalizations among super-utilizers than among other patients regardless of payer.

The most common reason for hospitalization across payers was to treat a medical condition; other less common types of stays were surgical, mental health, injury, and maternal/neonatal. Medical stays were more common among super-utilizers than among other patients across all expected payers. The difference was most striking for privately insured and Medicaid patients—the share of medical stays among super-utilizers was nearly twice as high as among other patients (private insurance: 65.1 vs. 33.3 percent; Medicaid: 67.0 vs. 35.3 percent).

Mental health stays also were more common for super-utilizers than for other patients among privately insured (7.7 vs. 5.7 percent) and Medicaid patients (19.3 vs. 11.6 percent.)

Resource use and outcomes of hospital stays for super-utilizers by payer, 2012.

Figure 1 presents the share of total hospital stays, hospital days, hospital costs, and readmissions that were attributable to super-utilizers by payer in 2012.

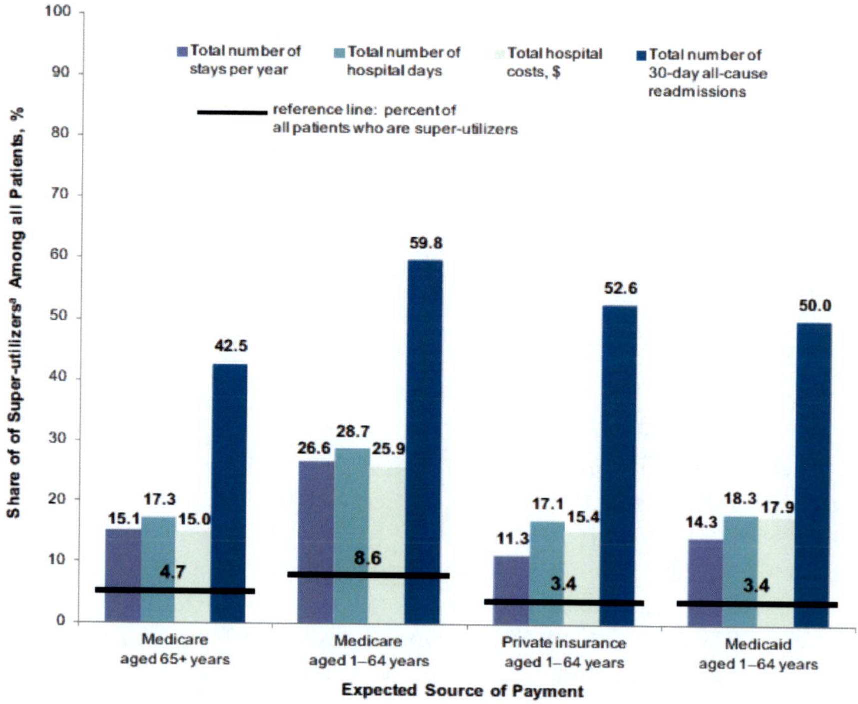

Source: Weighted national estimates from the Agency for Healthcare Research and Quality (AHRQ), Center for Delivery, Organization, and Markets, Healthcare Cost and Utilization Project (HCUP), Nationwide Readmissions Database (NRD), 2012.

[a] Super-utilizers are Medicare and Medicaid patients with four or more hospital stays and privately insured patients with three or more hospital stays in 2012.

Figure 1. Share of resource use and outcomes for super-utilizersa among all patients by payer, 2012.

- Super-utilizers accounted for a disproportionate share of hospital stays, days, costs, and all cause 30-day readmissions compared with other patients.

As indicated by the reference line in Figure 1, there were relatively few super-utilizers in 2012—they constituted only 4.7 percent of hospitalized Medicare patients aged 65+ years, 8.6 percent of hospitalized Medicare patients aged 1–64 years, 3.4 percent of hospitalized privately insured patients, and 3.4 percent of hospitalized Medicaid patients. However, across all payers, super-utilizers accounted for a substantially higher proportion of hospital stays, days, costs, and all-cause 30-day readmissions. For example, although only 4.7 percent of hospitalized Medicare patients aged 65 years and older were super-utilizers, they accounted for more than three times as many hospitals stays (15.1 percent), hospital days (17.3 percent), and hospital costs (15.0 percent), and more than nine times as many readmissions (42.5 percent). The disproportionate share of resources used by super-utilizers was most pronounced for readmissions. Among privately insured and Medicaid patients, fewer than 4 percent (super-utilizers) accounted for about half of all hospital readmissions.

DATA SOURCE

The estimates in this Statistical Brief are based upon data from the Healthcare Cost and Utilization Project (HCUP) 2012 Nationwide Readmissions Database (NRD). The 2012 NRD is planned for public release in fall 2015. The NRD is a calendar-year, discharge-level database constructed from the HCUP State Inpatient Databases (SID) with verified patient linkage numbers that can be used to track a person across hospitals within a State. The NRD is designed to support various types of analyses of national readmission rates. The database includes discharges for patients with and without repeat hospital visits in a year and those who have died in the hospital. Repeat stays may or may not be related to one another. The criteria to determine the relationship between hospital admissions is left to the analyst using the NRD. The NRD was constructed as a sample of convenience consisting of 100 percent of the eligible discharges in HCUP States that provide the ability to link patients across hospital stays. Discharge weights for national estimates were developed using the target universe of community hospitals (excluding rehabilitation and long-term acute care hospitals) in the United States and poststratification on hospital characteristics (census region, urban-rural location, teaching status, bed size, and control/ownership) and patient age-sex groups. Only patients aged 1 year and older were included in the analysis. Verified patient linkage numbers tend to be less reliable and less complete for patients less than 1 year old, which makes it difficult to track multiple hospitalizations.

DEFINITIONS

Diagnoses, ICD-9-CM and Clinical Classifications Software (CCS)

The principal diagnosis is that condition established after study to be chiefly responsible for the patient's admission to the hospital.

ICD-9-CM is the International Classification of Diseases, Ninth Revision, Clinical Modification, which assigns numeric codes to diagnoses. There are approximately 14,000 ICD-9-CM diagnosis codes.

CCS categorizes ICD-9-CM diagnosis codes into a manageable number of clinically meaningful categories.[9] This clinical grouper makes it easier to quickly understand patterns of diagnoses. CCS categories identified as Other typically are not reported; these categories include miscellaneous, otherwise unclassifiable diagnoses that may be difficult to interpret as a group.

Types of hospitals included in the HCUP Nationwide Readmissions Database.

The Nationwide Readmissions Database (NRD) is based on data from community hospitals, which are defined as short-term, non-Federal, general, and other hospitals, excluding hospital units of other institutions (e.g., prisons). The NRD includes obstetrics and gynecology, otolaryngology, orthopedic, cancer, pediatric, public, and academic medical hospitals. Excluded are long-term care facilities such as rehabilitation, longterm acute care, psychiatric, and alcoholism and chemical dependency hospitals. However, if a patient received long-term care, rehabilitation, or treatment for psychiatric or chemical dependency conditions in a community hospital, the discharge record for that stay will be included in the NRD.

Unit of Analysis

The unit of analysis is the hospital discharge (i.e., the hospital stay), not a person or patient. This means that a person who is admitted to the hospital multiple times in 1 year will be counted each time as a separate discharge from the hospital.

Hospital use in the year determined which category (e.g., Medicare super-utilizers aged 1–64 years) included all stays for a patient. The payer-age group for the patient was defined by the first hospital stay in the year. For example, a Medicare patient who was 64 years old for a January stay and 65 years old for

September hospital stay would be included in the group Medicare aged 1–64 years. After each patient was assigned to a payer-age group, the total number of hospital stays in 2012 was determined for each unique patient (based on the HCUP data element VisitLink). Using the distribution of total number of hospital stays within each payer-age group, the cut-off for super-utilizers was defined as approximately two standard deviations above the average total number of hospital stays. The assignment of the payer-age group and whether the patient qualified as a super-utilizer in that group was then added to each hospital stay discharge for that patient. The analysis considered all hospital stays in the year, with the exception of the counts of readmissions.

Readmissions

The 30-day readmission rate is defined as the number of admissions for each condition for which there was at least one subsequent hospital admission within 30 days, divided by the total number of admissions from January through November 2012. That is, when patients are discharged from the hospital, they are followed for 30 days in the data. If any readmission to the same or to a different hospital occurs during this time period, the admission is counted as a readmission. No more than one readmission is counted within the 30- day period of each admission, because the outcome measure assessed is the "percentage of admissions that are followed by a readmission." If a patient was transferred to a different hospital on the same day or was transferred within the same hospital, the two events were combined as a single stay and the second event was not counted as a readmission; that is, a transfer was not considered a readmission.

Costs and Charges

Total hospital charges were converted to costs using HCUP Cost-to-Charge Ratios based on hospital accounting reports from the Centers for Medicare & Medicaid Services (CMS).[10] *Costs* reflect the actual expenses incurred in the production of hospital services, such as wages, supplies, and utility costs; *charges* represent the amount a hospital billed for the case. For each hospital, a hospital-wide cost-to-charge ratio is used. Hospital charges reflect the amount the hospital billed for the entire hospital stay and do not include professional (physician) fees. For the purposes of this Statistical Brief, costs are reported to the nearest hundred.

How HCUP estimates of costs differ from National Health Expenditure Accounts.

There are a number of differences between the costs cited in this Statistical Brief and spending as measured in the National Health Expenditure Accounts (NHEA), which are produced annually by CMS.[11] The largest source of difference comes from the HCUP coverage of inpatient treatment only in contrast to the NHEA inclusion of outpatient costs associated with emergency departments and other hospital-based outpatient clinics and departments as well. The outpatient portion of hospitals' activities has been growing steadily and may exceed half of all hospital revenue in recent years. On the basis of the American Hospital Association Annual Survey, 2012 outpatient gross revenues (or charges) were about 44 percent of total hospital gross revenues.[12]

Smaller sources of differences come from the inclusion in the NHEA of hospitals that are excluded from HCUP. These include Federal hospitals (Department of Defense, Veterans Administration, Indian Health Services, and Department of Justice [prison] hospitals) as well as psychiatric, substance abuse, and longterm care hospitals. A third source of difference lies in the HCUP reliance on billed charges from hospitals to payers, adjusted to provide estimates of costs using hospital-wide cost-to-charge ratios, in contrast to the NHEA measurement of spending or revenue. HCUP costs estimate the amount of money required to produce hospital services, including expenses for wages, salaries, and benefits paid to staff as well as utilities, maintenance, and other similar expenses required to run a hospital. NHEA spending or revenue measures the amount of income received by the hospital for treatment and other services provided, including payments by insurers, patients, or government programs. The difference between revenues and costs include profit for for-profit hospitals or surpluses for nonprofit hospitals.

Payer

Payer is the expected primary payer for the hospital stay. To make coding uniform across all HCUP data sources, payer combines detailed categories into general groups:

- Medicare: includes patients covered by fee-for-service and managed care Medicare.

- Medicaid: includes patients covered by fee-for-service and managed care Medicaid.
- Private Insurance: includes Blue Cross, commercial carriers, and private health maintenance organizations (HMOs) and preferred provider organizations (PPOs).
- Uninsured: includes an insurance status of *self-pay* and *no charge*
- Other: includes Worker's Compensation, TRICARE/CHAMPUS, CHAMPVA, Title V, and other government programs.

Hospital stays billed to the State Children's Health Insurance Program (SCHIP) may be classified as Medicaid, Private Insurance, or Other, depending on the structure of the State program. Because most State data do not identify patients in SCHIP specifically, it is not possible to present this information separately.

For the purpose of this analysis, the expected payer designation was assigned based on a hierarchy of Medicare, Medicaid, and then privately insured. Medicare was identified based on a payer code of Medicare as a primary, secondary, or tertiary payer regardless of any other reported payers. This means that individuals who were dually eligible for Medicare and Medicaid were categorized as Medicare. If not already assigned to Medicare, Medicaid was identified based on a payer code of Medicaid as a primary, secondary, or tertiary payer regardless of any other reported payers. If not already assigned to Medicare or Medicaid, private insurance was identified based on a payer code of private insurance as a primary, secondary, or tertiary payer.

About HCUP

The Healthcare Cost and Utilization Project (HCUP, pronounced "H-Cup") is a family of health care databases and related software tools and products developed through a Federal-State-Industry partnership and sponsored by the Agency for Healthcare Research and Quality (AHRQ). HCUP databases bring together the data collection efforts of State data organizations, hospital associations, and private data organizations (HCUP Partners) and the Federal government to create a national information resource of encounter-level health care data. HCUP includes the largest collection of longitudinal hospital care data in the United States, with all-payer, encounter-level information beginning in 1988. These databases enable research on a broad range of health policy issues, including cost and quality of health services, medical practice patterns, access to health care programs, and outcomes of treatments at the national, State, and local market levels.

HCUP would not be possible without the contributions of the following data collection Partners from across the United States:

Alaska State Hospital and Nursing Home Association
Arizona Department of Health Services
Arkansas Department of Health
California Office of Statewide Health Planning and Development
Colorado Hospital Association
Connecticut Hospital Association
District of Columbia Hospital Association
Florida Agency for Health Care Administration
Georgia Hospital Association
Hawaii Health Information Corporation
Illinois Department of Public Health
Indiana Hospital Association
Iowa Hospital Association
Kansas Hospital Association
Kentucky Cabinet for Health and Family Services
Louisiana Department of Health and Hospitals
Maine Health Data Organization
Maryland Health Services Cost Review Commission
Massachusetts Center for Health Information and Analysis
Michigan Health & Hospital Association
Minnesota Hospital Association
Mississippi Department of Health
Missouri Hospital Industry Data Institute
Montana MHA - An Association of Montana Health Care Providers
Nebraska Hospital Association
Nevada Department of Health and Human Services
New Hampshire Department of Health & Human Services
New Jersey Department of Health
New Mexico Department of Health
New York State Department of Health
North Carolina Department of Health and Human Services
North Dakota (data provided by the Minnesota Hospital Association)

Ohio Hospital Association
Oklahoma State Department of Health
Oregon Association of Hospitals and Health Systems
Oregon Office of Health Analytics
Pennsylvania Health Care Cost Containment Council
Rhode Island Department of Health
South Carolina Revenue and Fiscal Affairs Office
South Dakota Association of Healthcare Organizations
Tennessee Hospital Association
Texas Department of State Health Services
Utah Department of Health
Vermont Association of Hospitals and Health Systems
Virginia Health Information
Washington State Department of Health
West Virginia Health Care Authority
Wisconsin Department of Health Services
Wyoming Hospital Association

About Statistical Briefs

HCUP Statistical Briefs are descriptive summary reports presenting statistics on hospital inpatient and emergency department use and costs, quality of care, access to care, medical conditions, procedures, patient populations, and other topics. The reports use HCUP administrative health care data.

About the NRD

The HCUP Nationwide Readmissions Database (NRD) is a calendar-year, discharge-level database constructed from the HCUP State Inpatient Databases (SID) with verified patient linkage numbers that can be used to track a person across hospitals within a State. The 2012 NRD is planned for public release in fall 2015. The NRD is designed to support various types of analyses of national readmission rates. The database includes discharges for patients with and without repeat hospital visits in a year and those who have died in the hospital. Repeat stays may or may not be related. The criteria to determine the relationship between hospital admissions is left to the analyst using the NRD. The NRD was constructed as a sample of convenience consisting of 100 percent of the eligible discharges. Discharge weights for national estimates are developed using the target universe of community hospitals (excluding rehabilitation and long-term acute care hospitals) in the United States.

For More Information

For more information about HCUP, visit http://www.hcup-us.ahrq.gov/.

For additional HCUP statistics, visit HCUPnet, our interactive query system, at http://hcupnet.ahrq.gov/. HCUPnet provides ready-to-use tables on readmission rates by condition and procedure (using Clinical Classification Software categories), diagnosis-related groups (DRGs), and major diagnostic categories (MDCs).

For information on readmissions-related topics, refer to the following HCUP Statistical Briefs located at http://www.hcup-us.ahrq.gov/reports/statbriefs/statbriefs.jsp:

- Statistical Brief #184, Characteristics of Hospital Stays for Nonelderly Medicaid Super-Utilizers, 2012.
- Statistical Brief #172, Conditions With the Largest Number of Adult Hospital Readmissions by Payer, 2011.
- Statistical Brief #127, 30-Day Readmissions following Hospitalizations for Chronic vs. Acute Conditions, 2008.
- Statistical Brief #115, All-Cause Readmissions by Payer and Age, 2008.
- Statistical Brief #89, All-Cause Hospital Readmissions among Non-Elderly Medicaid Patients, 2007.

End Notes

[1] Stanton MW, Rutherford MK. The high concentration of U.S. health care expenditures. Research in Action Issue 19. 2005. Rockville, MD: Agency for Healthcare Research and Quality. http://meps.ahrq.gov/mepsweb/datafiles/publications/ra19/ra19.pdf. Accessed February 5, 2015.

[2] Ibid.

[3] Gawande A. The hot spotters: can we lower medical costs by giving the neediest patients better care? The New Yorker. January 24, 2011. http://www.newyorker.com/magazine/2011/01/24/the-hot-spotters. Accessed February 20, 2015.

[4] Emeche U. Is a strategy focused on super-utilizers equal to the task of health care system transformation? Yes. Annals of Family Medicine. 2015;13(1):6–7.

[5] Robert Wood Johnson Foundation. A Revolutionary Approach to Improving Health Care Delivery. Better Care for Super-Utilizers series. February 1, 2014. http://www.rwjf.org/en/about-rwjf/newsroom/newsroom-content/2012/10/improvingmanagement-of-health-care-superutilizers.html. Accessed April 13, 2015.

[6] Jiang HJ, Barrett ML, Sheng M. Characteristics of Hospital Stays for Nonelderly Medicaid Super-utilizers, 2012. HCUP Statistical Brief #184. November 2014. Rockville, MD: Agency for Healthcare Research and Quality. http://www.hcup-us.ahrq.gov/reports/statbriefs/sb184-Hospital-Stays-Medicaid-Super-Utilizers-2012.pdf. Accessed February 5, 2015.

[7] Ibid.

[8] Four or more hospital stays for Medicare and Medicaid patients and three or more hospital stays for privately insured patients are approximately two standard deviations above the average number of hospital stays for patients in each payer category.

[9] Agency for Healthcare Research and Quality. HCUP Clinical Classifications Software (CCS). Healthcare Cost and Utilization Project (HCUP). Rockville, MD: Agency for Healthcare Research and Quality. Updated November 2014. http://www.hcup-us.ahrq.gov/tools software/ccs/ccs.jsp. Accessed January 7, 2015.

[10] Agency for Healthcare Research and Quality. HCUP Cost-to-Charge Ratio (CCR) Files. Healthcare Cost and Utilization Project (HCUP). 2001–2012. Rockville, MD: Agency for Healthcare Research and Quality. Updated December 2014. http://www.hcupus.ahrq.gov/db/state/costtocharge.jsp. Accessed January 7, 2015.

[11] For additional information about the NHEA, see Centers for Medicare & Medicaid Services (CMS). National Health Expenditure Data. CMS Web site May 2014. http://www.cms.gov/Research-Statistics-Data-and-Systems/Statistics-Trends-and-Reports/NationalHealthExpendData/index.html?redirect=/NationalHealthExpendData/. Accessed January 7, 2015.

[12] American Hospital Association. TrendWatch Chartbook, 2014. Table 4.2. Distribution of Inpatient vs. Outpatient Revenues, 1992–2012. http://www.aha.org/research/reports/tw/chartbook/2014/table4-2.pdf. Accessed January 7, 2015.

In: Significant Health Statistics
Editor: Christopher Barrett
ISBN: 978-1-63484-563-2

Chapter 5

TRENDS IN HOSPITAL READMISSIONS FOR FOUR HIGH-VOLUME CONDITIONS, 2009–2013*

Kathryn Fingar, PhD, MPH and Raynard Washington, PhD

HIGHLIGHTS

- In 2013, there were about 500,000 readmissions totaling $7 billion in aggregate hospital costs for four high-volume conditions—acute myocardial infarction (AMI), congestive heart failure (CHF), chronic obstructive pulmonary disease (COPD), and pneumonia.
- Among initial hospital stays (*index stays*) for AMI, CHF, COPD, and pneumonia, the aggregate cost of readmissions in 2013 was $5.2 billion for Medicare—74 percent of the aggregate cost of readmissions for these four conditions.
- From 2009 to 2013, the readmission rate for stays covered by Medicare decreased by 13 percent for AMI, by 7 percent each for CHF and COPD, and by 6 percent for pneumonia.

---

* This is an edited, reformatted and augmented version of Healthcare Cost and Utilization Project (HCUP) Statistical Brief #196, issued by the Agency for Healthcare Research and Quality, November 2015.

- Overall, the largest decrease in readmission rate from 2009 to 2013 was for AMI (by 13 percent, from 16.9 to 14.7 readmissions per 100 index stays for AMI). Although the rate declined overall (across payers), the aggregate cost of readmissions following an index stay for AMI decreased only among index stays covered by private insurance (by 18 percent).
- Although Medicare was the only payer for which the rate of readmission for pneumonia decreased from 2009 to 2013, the aggregate cost of readmissions for pneumonia decreased for all payers, by 6–26 percent.
- The aggregate cost of readmissions following an index stay for any of the four conditions decreased from 2009 to 2013 for all payers, except the uninsured whose rate remain unchanged. The largest declines were for index stays paid by private insurance (22 percent) and Medicare (9 percent).

INTRODUCTION

Hospital readmissions can have negative consequences for patients and the hospitals at which they are treated, and also are costly for both public and private payers. In 2011, Medicare paid for 58 percent of all readmissions, followed by private insurance (20 percent) and Medicaid (18 percent).[1] Readmissions are a significant portion of Medicare spending—37 percent of total Medicare spending is for inpatient care, and 18 percent of all inpatient admissions paid by Medicare are readmitted within 30 days, accounting for $15 billion in costs annually.[2] In addition to these costs, repeat hospitalizations place patients at greater risk for complications, hospital acquired infections, and stress.[3] Because the majority of readmissions are for nonsurgical services, it is unlikely that readmissions are profitable for hospitals.[4]

Although it may be necessary to readmit some patients, the fact that risk-adjusted readmission rates vary considerably across hospitals suggests that certain readmissions may be prevented through hospital practices, such as improving patient discharge instructions, coordinating postacute care, and reducing medical complications during the initial hospital stay.[5]

The Affordable Care Act established the Centers for Medicare & Medicaid Services Hospital Readmissions Reduction Program (HRRP) to provide a financial incentive for hospitals to reduce preventable readmissions.

Effective in 2013, the HRRP imposes a financial penalty for hospitals with excess rates of readmissions for acute myocardial infarction (AMI), congestive heart failure (CHF), and pneumonia among Medicare beneficiaries. In 2015, penalties also will be calculated based on readmissions for chronic obstructive pulmonary disease (COPD) and hip and knee replacements.[6] CMS includes these conditions and procedures because of their high volume and costs.[7]

This Healthcare Cost and Utilization Project (HCUP) Statistical Brief examines trends from 2009 through 2013 for all readmissions following an admission for any cause, as well as for readmissions following an admission for four high-volume conditions targeted by the HRRP: AMI, CHF, COPD, and pneumonia. *Readmission* was defined as a subsequent hospital admission for any cause within 30 days following an initial hospital admission, referred to as the *index stay*. Because all-cause readmissions were examined, readmissions may or may not be related to the primary reason for admission during the index stay. Trends in the rate and aggregate cost of readmissions were examined overall and by expected payer of the index stay. Therefore, the expected payer of the readmission may be different from that of the index stay. Aggregate costs are those for the readmission only, not counting the cost of the index stay. Differences of greater than 5 percent are noted in the text.

FINDINGS

Readmission rates among high-volume conditions, 2013.

Table 1 presents conditions with at least 250,000 index stays that had the highest rate of readmission for all causes within 30 days in 2013. The four highlighted conditions—AMI, CHF, COPD, and pneumonia— are the focus of this Statistical Brief.

- AMI, CHF, COPD, and pneumonia accounted for 13 percent of all readmissions, as well as 13 percent of aggregate hospital costs for readmissions in 2013.

In 2013, there were 496,502 readmissions following an index stay for AMI, CHF, COPD, or pneumonia, accounting for 13 percent of all readmissions. Aggregate hospital costs for readmissions following an index stay for any of these four conditions totaled $7.0 billion—13 percent of aggregate costs for all readmissions.

Table 1. High-volume conditions ranked by rate of readmission for all causes within 30 days, 2013

Rank	Principal diagnosis for index hospital stay	Number of index admis-sions	Number of all-cause readmis-sions	Aggregate cost of readmis-sions, $ millions	Rate of all-cause readmission
Total index admissions for any cause		28,124,869	3,900,556	52,398	13.9
1	Congestive heart failure, non-hypertensive	782,079	183,534	2,728	23.5
2	Schizophrenia and other psychotic disorders	366,256	83,245	772	22.7
3	Respiratory failure, insufficiency, arrest (adult)	290,892	62,684	961	21.5
4	Diabetes mellitus with complications	486,886	99,108	1,204	20.4
5	Acute renal failure	431,452	87,537	1,190	20.3
6	Chronic obstructive pulmonary disease and bronchiectasis	570,077	114,067	1,384	20.0
7	Complication of device, implant or graft	581,289	111,838	1,973	19.2
8	Alcohol-related disorders	261,072	50,081	366	19.2
9	Septicemia	1,011,496	191,156	3,154	18.9
10	Fluid and electrolyte disorders	358,640	65,704	839	18.3
11	Complications of surgical procedures or medical care	426,917	76,292	1,212	17.9
12	Pancreatic disorders (not diabetes)	271,749	47,111	563	17.3
13	Gastrointestinal hemorrhage	328,428	55,173	741	16.8
14	Urinary tract infection	470,448	73,633	854	15.7
15	Intestinal obstruction without hernia	314,811	48,753	696	15.5
16	Pneumonia	824,700	127,601	1,809	15.5
17	Mood disorders	747,029	114,385	930	15.3
18	Acute myocardial infarction	485,462	71,300	1,043	14.7
19	Dysrhythmia	651,881	94,883	1,225	14.6
20	Coronary atherosclerosis and other heart disease	433,782	55,265	793	12.7

Source: Agency for Healthcare Research and Quality (AHRQ), Center for Delivery, Organization, and Markets, Healthcare Cost and Utilization Project (HCUP), Nationwide Readmissions Database (NRD), 2013.

Notes: Only conditions with greater than 250,000 index stays are shown. Principal diagnosis is based on the Clinical Classifications Software (CCS). Costs include those of the readmission only, excluding the cost of the index stay.

- Readmission rates for AMI, CHF, COPD, and pneumonia were more than 5 percent higher than the overall readmission rate of 13.9 per 100 index stays.

The rate of readmission following an index stay for CHF was the highest (23.5 per 100 index stays) among high-volume conditions with at least 250,000 index stays and was 69 percent higher than the rate of readmission overall (13.9). The rate of readmission was 20.0 per 100 index stays for COPD and 15.5 per 100 index stays for pneumonia—44 and 12 percent higher, respectively, than the rate of readmission overall. The rate of readmission for AMI (14.7) was 6 percent higher than the overall readmission rate in 2013.

Trends in readmissions for AMI, CHF, COPD, and pneumonia, 2009–2013.

Figure 1 presents trends in the rate of readmissions for any cause within 30 days, per 100 index stays, overall and for four high-volume conditions from 2009 through 2013.

- The percentage of index stays with AMI that were readmitted for any cause within 30 days decreased by 13 percent from 2009 through 2013.

From 2009 through 2013, the rate of readmission following index stays for AMI decreased by 13 percent, from 16.9 to 14.7 per 100 index stays. By 2013, the readmission rate following AMI was only 6 percent higher than the overall readmission rate of 13.9 per 100 index stays (vs. 21 percent higher in 2009).

- The rate of readmission for index stays with CHF or COPD decreased by 6 percent from 2009 through 2013.

From 2009 through 2013, the rate of readmission following index stays decreased by 6 percent for CHF (from 25.1 to 23.5 per 100 index stays) and for COPD (from 21.2 to 20.0 per 100 index stays).

The overall readmission rate and the readmission rate for pneumonia remained relatively stable from 2009 through 2013.

Table 2 presents trends in the 30-day all-cause readmission rate following index admissions for four high-volume conditions, by expected payer of the index stay, in 2009 and 2013.

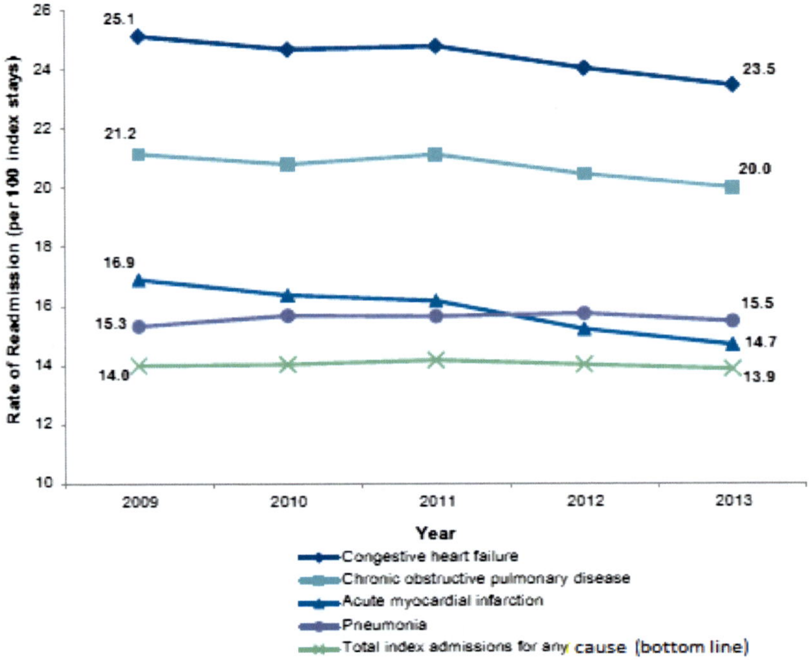

Source: Agency for Healthcare Research and Quality (AHRQ), Center for Delivery, Organization, and Markets, Healthcare Cost and Utilization Project (HCUP), 2013 Nationwide Readmissions Database (NRD), and weighted national estimates from readmissions analysis files derived from the 2009–2012 State Inpatient Databases (SID)

Note: Principal diagnosis grouped according to the Clinical Classifications Software (CCS)

Figure 1. All-cause rate of readmission, by principal diagnosis of index admission, 2009–2013.

Table 2. All-cause rate of readmission, by principal diagnosis and expected payer of the index stay, 2009–2013

Principal diagnosis for index hospital stay, by expected payer of the index stay	Number of all-cause readmissions		Rate of all-cause readmission		Cumulative percentage change in rate, 2009–2013
	2009	2013	2009	2013	
Total, all four conditions					
Total	571,393	496,502	19.7	18.6	–5.4

Principal diagnosis for index hospital stay, by expected payer of the index stay	Number of all-cause readmissions		Rate of all-cause readmission		Cumulative percentage change in rate, 2009–2013
	2009	2013	2009	2013	
Expected payer of index stay					
Medicare	430,916	376,761	22.0	20.3	−7.9
Medicaid	64,000	57,064	19.8	20.5	3.5
Private	54,824	40,350	12.4	11.7	−5.8
Uninsured	13,473	12,627	11.5	11.0	−4.0
Acute myocardial infarction					
Total	79,199	71,300	16.9	14.7	−13.1
Expected payer of index stay					
Medicare	56,348	51,334	20.4	17.8	−12.8
Medicaid	5,962	5,683	19.9	17.7	−10.7
Private	12,475	9,652	10.4	8.5	−18.3
Uninsured	2,953	3,011	9.8	8.6	−12.9
Congestive heart failure					
Total	214,198	183,534	25.1	23.5	−6.6
Expected payer of index stay					
Medicare	168,791	144,138	25.6	23.7	−7.2
Medicaid	22,285	19,809	30.4	29.1	−4.1
Private	16,309	11,973	19.8	18.3	−7.7
Uninsured	4,218	4,096	17.6	16.5	−6.4
Chronic obstructive pulmonary disease					
Total	132,098	114,067	21.2	20.0	−5.4
Expected payer of index stay					
Medicare	100,243	86,112	22.2	20.6	−7.3
Medicaid	17,405	16,053	24.1	24.5	1.7
Private	9,364	7,041	13.9	13.7	−1.1
Uninsured	3,038	2,594	13.9	12.0	−14.0
Pneumonia					
Total	145,898	127,601	15.3	15.5	1.0
Expected payer of index stay					
Medicare	105,534	95,178	18.6	17.5	−5.6
Medicaid	18,348	15,519	12.4	13.7	10.6
Private	16,676	11,685	9.6	10.1	4.8
Uninsured	3,263	2,926	7.9	8.9	13.3

Source: Agency for Healthcare Research and Quality (AHRQ), Center for Delivery, Organization, and Markets, Healthcare Cost and Utilization Project (HCUP), 2013 Nationwide Readmissions Database (NRD), and weighted national estimates from a readmissions analysis file derived from the 2009 State Inpatient Databases (SID).

Note: Principal diagnosis grouped according to the Clinical Classifications Software (CCS). Data by payer do not add to the column total because other payers are not shown.

- In 2009 and 2013, index stays paid by Medicare accounted for over 75 percent of readmissions for AMI, CHF, COPD, and pneumonia, and had higher readmission rates than any other payer, except for Medicaid.

Of all readmissions following an index stay for AMI, CHF, COPD, or pneumonia, over 75 percent had Medicare as the expected payer for the index stay in both 2009 and 2013. The rate of readmission for any of these four high-volume conditions among index stays with Medicare as the expected payer was nearly twice the rate among index stays with private insurance (20.3 vs. 11.7 per 100 index stays in 2013). In 2013, the rate of readmission for these four conditions also was high among index stays with Medicaid (20.5); it was lowest among uninsured index stays (11.0).

- The total rate of readmission associated with index stays for any of the four conditions examined decreased for all payers, except index stays paid by Medicaid.

The readmission rate among index stays for AMI, CHF, COPD, and pneumonia combined decreased by 7.9 percent for index stays paid by Medicare and by 5.8 percent for index stays paid by private insurance. The rate also decreased among uninsured index stays, although not by more than 5 percent. Medicaid was the only payer for which the readmission rate did not decrease from 2009 through 2013.

- The readmission rate decreased by more than 5 percent for each of the four high-volume conditions for index stays paid by Medicare.

From 2009 through 2013, among index stays with Medicare as the expected payer, the rate of readmission decreased by 13 percent for AMI, by 7 percent each for CHF and COPD, and by 6 percent for pneumonia. Medicare was the only expected payer for which the rate of readmission decreased for all four conditions.

- From 2009 through 2013, the rate of readmission following an index stay for AMI decreased by over 10 percent for all expected payers.

Private payers experienced the greatest decrease in the rate of readmission associated with AMI, by 18 percent, from 10.4 readmissions per 100 index stays in 2009 to 8.5 per 100 index stays in 2013. The rate of readmission following AMI decreased by 13 percent among index stays covered by Medicare and among uninsured index stays, and by 11 percent among index stays covered by Medicaid.

- The rate of readmission following an index stay for CHF decreased by over 5 percent for all expected payers except Medicaid.

The rate of readmission for CHF decreased by 8 percent among index stays covered by private insurance, by 7 percent among index stays with Medicare, and by 6 percent among uninsured index stays. The decrease in the CHF readmission rate was less than 5 percent for Medicaid.

- From 2009 through 2013, the rate of readmission following an index stay for pneumonia increased by 13 percent for uninsured stays and by 11 percent for stays covered by Medicaid.

The rate of readmission following an index stay for pneumonia remained stable at around 15.5 per 100 index stays overall. However, of the four high-volume conditions examined, pneumonia was the only condition for which the readmission rate increased by over 5 percent for any payer. This increase was highest among uninsured index stays, from 7.9 readmissions per 100 index stays in 2009 to 8.9 per 100 index stays in 2013 (a 13 percent increase), followed by index stays with Medicaid as the expected payer (an 11 percent increase). Medicare was the only payer for which the readmission rate associated with pneumonia decreased (by 6 percent).

Figure 2 presents the inflation-adjusted aggregate costs for readmissions for four high-volume conditions, by expected payer of the index stay, from 2009 through 2013.

- In 2013, the aggregate cost of readmissions for AMI, CHF, COPD, and pneumonia totaled $5.2 billion among index stays with Medicare.

Among index stays for AMI, CHF, COPD, and pneumonia with Medicare as the expected payer, the aggregate cost of readmissions, excluding the cost of the index stay, totaled $5.2 billion, more than 6 times the aggregate cost of readmissions for index stays with Medicaid or private insurance.

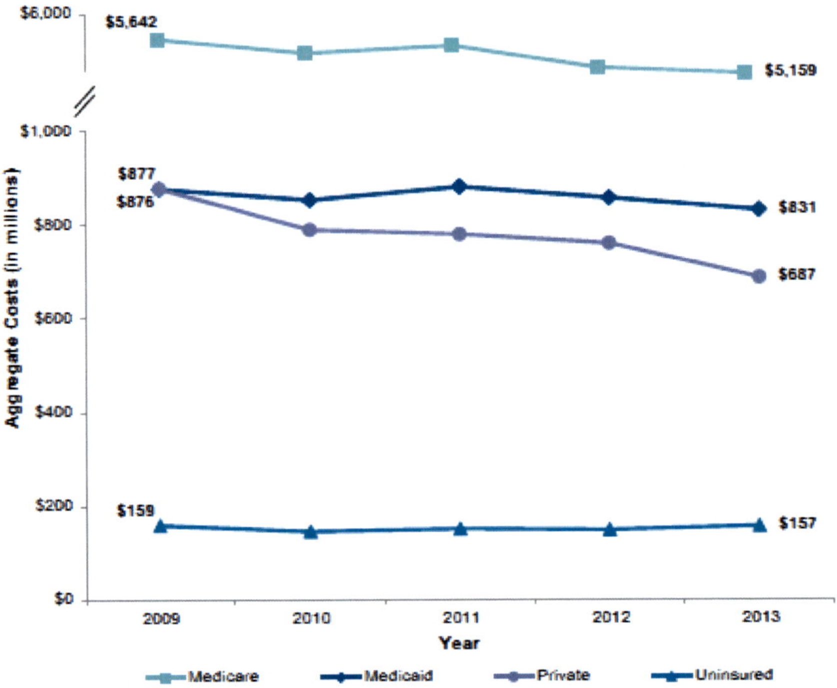

Source: Agency for Healthcare Research and Quality (AHRQ), Center for Delivery, Organization, and Markets, Healthcare Cost and Utilization Project (HCUP), 2013 Nationwide Readmissions Database (NRD), and weighted national estimates from readmissions analysis files derived from the 2009–2012 State Inpatient Databases (SID).

Abbreviations: AMI, acute myocardial infarction; CHF, congestive heart failure; COPD, chronic obstructive pulmonary disease.

Notes: All costs are inflation adjusted using the price index for the gross domestic product and expressed in 2013 dollars. Costs include those of the readmission only, excluding the cost of the index stay.

Figure 2. Inflation-adjusted aggregate costs for readmissions for any cause following an index stay for AMI, CHF, COPD, or pneumonia, by expected payer of the index stay, 2009–2013.

- Overall, the aggregate cost of readmissions following an index stay for any of the four conditions decreased for all payers. The largest declines were among index stays paid by private insurance (22 percent) and by Medicare (9 percent).

From 2009 through 2013, the inflation-adjusted aggregate cost of readmissions among index stays for AMI, CHF, COPD, and pneumonia that were expected to be paid by private insurance decreased 22 percent, from $877 to $687 million. The aggregate cost of readmissions for these four conditions over the 5-year time period also decreased among index stays paid by Medicare (by 9 percent from $5,642 to $5,159 million) and among index stays paid by Medicaid (by 5 percent from $876 to $831 million). Aggregate costs remained relatively stable for uninsured index stays, decreasing by less than 5 percent.

Table 3 presents inflation-adjusted aggregate costs for readmissions for four high-volume conditions, by principal diagnosis and expected payer of the index stay, in 2009 and 2013.

Table 3. Inflation-adjusted aggregate costs of readmissions for four high-volume conditions, by principal diagnosis and expected payer of the index stay, 2009–2013

Principal diagnosis for index hospital stay, by expected payer of the index stay	Aggregate costs for readmissions, $ millions		Cumulative percentage change in aggregate costs, 2009–2013
	2009	2013	
Total, all four conditions			
Total	7,661.6	6,964.7	–9.1
Expected payer of index stay			
Medicare	5,642.3	5,158.6	–8.6
Medicaid	876.5	831.3	–5.2
Private	877.4	687.1	–21.7
Uninsured	159.2	156.8	–1.5
Acute myocardial infarction			
Total	1,098.3	1,043.4	–5.0
Expected payer of index stay			
Medicare	771.1	743.2	–3.6
Medicaid	83.8	86.9	3.6
Private	183.7	151.5	–17.6
Uninsured	38.2	39.7	4.0
Congestive heart failure			
Total	2,975.0	2,728.2	–8.3
Expected payer of index stay			
Medicare	2,249.6	2,055.9	–8.6
Medicaid	322.3	314.8	–2.3

Table 3. (Continued)

Principal diagnosis for index hospital stay, by expected payer of the index stay	Aggregate costs for readmissions, $ millions		Cumulative percentage change in aggregate costs, 2009–2013
	2009	2013	
Private	317.0	252.4	–20.4
Uninsured	50.9	56.2	10.4
Chronic obstructive pulmonary disease			
Total	1,572.3	1,383.6	–12.0
Expected payer of index stay			
Medicare	1,202.0	1,049.4	–12.7
Medicaid	198.3	189.2	–4.6
Private	120.2	94.3	–21.6
Uninsured	30.1	23.2	–22.9
Pneumonia			
Total	2,016.0	1,809.5	–10.2
Expected payer of index stay			
Medicare	1,419.6	1,310.1	–7.7
Medicaid	272.1	240.5	–11.6
Private	256.5	188.9	–26.4
Uninsured	40.0	37.7	–5.7

Source: Agency for Healthcare Research and Quality (AHRQ), Center for Delivery, Organization, and Markets, Healthcare Cost and Utilization Project (HCUP), 2013 Nationwide Readmissions Database (NRD), and weighted national estimates from a readmissions analysis file derived from the 2009 State Inpatient Databases (SID).

Notes: Principal diagnosis grouped according to the Clinical Classifications Software (CCS). All costs are inflation adjusted using the price index for the gross domestic product and expressed in 2013 dollars. Costs include those of the readmission only, excluding the cost of the index stay. Data by payer do not add to the column total because other payers are not shown.

- The aggregate cost of readmissions following an index stay for AMI decreased by 18 percent for index stays paid by private insurance.

The inflation-adjusted aggregate cost of readmissions following index stays for AMI with private insurance as the expected payer decreased from $183.7 to $151.5 million from 2009 through 2013 (by 18 percent). The aggregate cost of readmissions associated with AMI did not change by more than 5 percent for other expected payers.

- The aggregate cost of readmissions for CHF decreased by 20 percent among index stays paid by private insurance and by 9 percent among those paid by Medicare.

From 2009 through 2013, the aggregate cost of readmissions following an index stay for CHF decreased by 20 percent among index stays with private insurance as the expected payer (from $317.0 to $252.4 million) and by 9 percent among index stays with Medicare as the expected payer (from $2,249.6 to $2,055.9 million). By contrast, aggregate costs for readmissions following an index stay for CHF increased by 10 percent among index stays with no insurance (from $50.9 to $56.2 million).

- From 2009 through 2013, the aggregate cost of readmissions for COPD decreased by over 5 percent among all expected payers except Medicaid.

The aggregate cost of readmissions following an index stay for COPD decreased by 23 percent among uninsured index stays, by 22 percent among index stays with private insurance as the expected payer, and by 13 percent among index stays with Medicare as the expected payer. There was no substantial change in the aggregate cost of readmissions following index stays for COPD with Medicaid.

- The aggregate cost of readmissions for pneumonia decreased by over 5 percent among all expected payers.

The aggregate cost of readmissions following an index stay for pneumonia decreased for all expected payers: by 26 percent among index stays paid by private insurance, by 12 percent among index stays paid by Medicaid, by 8 percent among index stays paid by Medicare, and by 6 percent among uninsured index stays.

- Aggregate costs of readmissions following an index stay with private insurance decreased by more than 17 percent for each of the four high-volume conditions examined.

The aggregate cost of readmissions following an index stay with private insurance as the expected payer decreased between 18 and 26 percent for each of the four conditions examined (decrease of 18 percent for AMI, 20 percent for CHF, 22 percent for COPD, and 26 percent for pneumonia).

Data Source

The estimates in this Statistical Brief are based upon data from the Healthcare Cost and Utilization Project (HCUP) 2013 Nationwide Readmissions Database (NRD) and the 2009–2012 State Inpatient Databases (SID). The SID were used to create readmissions analysis files consistent with the design of the 2013 NRD and weighted for national estimates. The statistics were generated from HCUPnet, a free, online query system that provides users with *immediate access* to the largest set of publicly available, all-payer national, regional, and State-level hospital care databases from HCUP.[8]

Definitions

Diagnoses, ICD-9-CM, and Clinical Classifications Software (CCS).

The principal diagnosis is that condition established after study to be chiefly responsible for the patient's admission to the hospital. Secondary diagnoses are concomitant conditions that coexist at the time of admission or develop during the stay.

ICD-9-CM is the International Classification of Diseases, Ninth Revision, Clinical Modification, which assigns numeric codes to diagnoses. There are approximately 14,000 ICD-9-CM diagnosis codes.

CCS categorizes ICD-9-CM diagnosis codes into a manageable number of clinically meaningful categories.[9] This clinical grouper makes it easier to quickly understand patterns of diagnoses. CCS categories identified as Other typically are not reported; these categories include miscellaneous, otherwise unclassifiable diagnoses that may be difficult to interpret as a group.

High-Volume Conditions

The four high-volume conditions examined in this Statistical Brief were identified using the following CCS codes based on the principal diagnosis:

- Acute myocardial infarction (AMI): CCS 100
- Congestive heart failure (CHF): CCS 108
- Chronic obstructive pulmonary disease (COPD): CCS 127
- Pneumonia: CCS 122

These conditions were chosen because they are used to calculate readmission rates and penalty payment adjustments by the Centers for Medicare & Medicaid Services (CMS) Hospital Readmissions Reduction Program (HRRP). The HRRP also considers readmissions for index stays involving hip and knee replacements, which we did not examine in this Statistical Brief because these types of stays are identified using procedure rather than diagnosis codes.

It should be noted that our estimates may differ from Medicare readmission rates computed using other data sources. The CMS HRRP uses a different algorithm to identify conditions.[10] There may also be differences in the inclusion of beneficiaries with Medicare fee-for-service or Medicare Advantage and beneficiaries dually enrolled in Medicare and Medicaid. These groups are included in the Medicare estimates in this Statistical Brief. As shown in Table 4, despite these potential differences the rates of readmission following index stays for AMI, CHF, and pneumonia that were expected to be paid by Medicare, as reported in this Statistical Brief using HCUP data, are consistent with an analysis conducted by the Kaiser Family Foundation[11] using CMS Hospital Compare data (the latter did not report COPD readmission rates).

Readmissions

The 30-day readmission rate is defined as the number of admissions for each condition for which there was at least one subsequent hospital admission within 30 days, divided by the total number of admissions from January through November of the same year. That is, when patients are discharged from the hospital, they are followed for 30 days in the data.

If any readmission to the same or different hospital occurs during this time period, the admission is counted as having a readmission. No more than one readmission is counted within the 30-day period, because the outcome measure assessed is “percentage of admissions that are readmitted.” If a patient was transferred to a different hospital on the same day or was transferred within the same hospital, the two events were combined as a single stay and the second event was not counted as a readmission; that is, transfers were not considered a readmission. In the case of admissions for which there was more than one readmission in the 30-day period, the data presented in this Statistical Brief reflect the characteristics and costs of the first readmission.

Table 4. A comparison of Medicare readmission rates following index stays for AMI, CHF, and pneumonia for 2008–2013 published by the Kaiser Family Foundation with those for 2009 and 2013 from HCUP

Condition	KFF national average Medicare readmission rate, %		HCUP national Medicare readmission rate, %	
	2008–2011	2010–2013	2009	2013
AMI	19.7	17.8	20.4	17.8
CHF	24.7	22.7	25.6	23.7
Pneumonia	18.5	17.3	18.6	17.5

Source: Kaiser Family Foundation analysis of Centers for Medicare & Medicaid Services Hospital Compare data files; Agency for Healthcare Research and Quality (AHRQ), Center for Delivery, Organization, and Markets, Healthcare Cost and Utilization Project (HCUP), 2013 Nationwide Readmissions Database (NRD), and weighted national estimates from a readmissions analysis file derived from the 2009 State Inpatient Databases (SID).

Abbreviations: AMI, acute myocardial infarction; CHF, congestive heart failure; KFF, Kaiser Family Foundation.

Every qualifying hospital stay is counted as a separate initial (starting point) admission. Thus, a single patient can be counted multiple times during the course of the January through November observation period. In addition, initial admissions do not require a prior "clean period" with no hospitalizations; that is, a hospital stay may be a readmission for a prior stay and the initial admission for a subsequent readmission. Admissions were disqualified from the analysis as initial admissions if they could not be followed for 30 days for one of the following reasons: (1) the patient died in the hospital, (2) information on length of stay was missing, or (3) the patient was discharged in December.

Types of Hospitals Included in the HCUP Nationwide Readmissions Database

The Nationwide Readmissions Database (NRD) is based on data from community hospitals, which are defined as short-term, non-Federal, general, and other hospitals, excluding hospital units of other institutions (e.g., prisons). The NRD includes obstetrics and gynecology, otolaryngology, orthopedic, cancer, pediatric, public, and academic medical hospitals. Excluded are long-term care facilities such as rehabilitation, long-term acute care, psychiatric, and alcoholism and chemical dependency hospitals. However, if a patient received long-term care, rehabilitation, or treatment for psychiatric or chemical dependency conditions in a community hospital, the discharge record for that stay will be included in the NRD.

Types of Hospitals Included in HCUP State Inpatient Databases

This analysis used State Inpatient Databases (SID) limited to data from community hospitals, which are defined as short-term, non-Federal, general, and other hospitals, excluding hospital units of other institutions (e.g., prisons). Community hospitals include obstetrics and gynecology, otolaryngology, orthopedic, cancer, pediatric, public, and academic medical hospitals. Excluded for this analysis are long-term care facilities such as rehabilitation, psychiatric, and alcoholism and chemical dependency hospitals. However, if a patient received long-term care, rehabilitation, or treatment for psychiatric or chemical dependency conditions in a community hospital, the discharge record for that stay was included in the analysis.

Costs and Charges

Total hospital charges were converted to costs using HCUP Cost-to-Charge Ratios based on hospital accounting reports from CMS.[12] *Costs* reflect the actual expenses incurred in the production of hospital services, such as wages, supplies, and utility costs; *charges* represent the amount a hospital billed for the case. For each hospital, a hospital-wide cost-to-charge ratio is used. Hospital charges reflect the amount the hospital billed for the entire hospital stay and do not include professional (physician) fees. For the purposes of this Statistical Brief, costs are reported to the nearest hundred thousand.

Annual costs were inflation adjusted using the Gross Domestic Product (GDP) Price Index from the U.S. Department of Commerce, Bureau of Economic Analysis (BEA), with 2013 as the index base.[13] That is, all costs are expressed in 2013 dollars.

How HCUP Estimates of Costs Differ from National Health Expenditure Accounts

There are a number of differences between the costs cited in this Statistical Brief and spending as measured in the National Health Expenditure Accounts (NHEA), which are produced annually by CMS.[14] The largest source of difference comes from the HCUP coverage of inpatient treatment only in contrast to the NHEA inclusion of outpatient costs associated with emergency departments and other hospital-based outpatient clinics and departments as well. The outpatient portion of hospitals' activities has been growing steadily and may exceed half of all hospital revenue in recent years. On the basis of the American Hospital Association Annual Survey, 2012 outpatient gross revenues (or charges) were about 44 percent of total hospital gross revenues.[15]

Smaller sources of differences come from the inclusion in the NHEA of hospitals that are excluded from HCUP. These include Federal hospitals (Department of Defense, Veterans Administration, Indian Health Services, and Department of Justice [prison] hospitals) as well as psychiatric, substance abuse, and longterm care hospitals. A third source of difference lies in the HCUP reliance on billed charges from hospitals to payers, adjusted to provide estimates of costs using hospital-wide cost-to-charge ratios, in contrast to the NHEA measurement of spending or revenue. HCUP costs estimate the amount of money required to produce hospital services, including expenses for wages, salaries, and benefits paid to staff as well as utilities, maintenance, and other similar expenses required to run a hospital. NHEA spending or revenue measures the amount of income received by the hospital for treatment and other services provided, including payments by insurers, patients, or government programs. The difference between revenues and costs include profit for for-profit hospitals or surpluses for nonprofit hospitals.

Payer

Payer is the expected payer for the hospital stay. To make coding uniform across all HCUP data sources, payer combines detailed categories into general groups:

- Medicare: includes patients covered by fee-for-service and managed care Medicare.
- Medicaid: includes patients covered by fee-for-service and managed care Medicaid.
- Private Insurance: includes Blue Cross, commercial carriers, and private health maintenance organizations (HMOs) and preferred provider organizations (PPOs).
- Uninsured: includes an insurance status of self-pay and no charge.
- Other: includes Worker's Compensation, TRICARE/CHAMPUS, CHAMPVA, Title V, and other government programs.

Hospital stays billed to the State Children's Health Insurance Program (SCHIP) may be classified as Medicaid, Private Insurance, or Other, depending on the structure of the State program. Because most State data do not identify SCHIP patients specifically, it is not possible to present this information separately.

For this Statistical Brief a hierarchy was used to assign the payer category based on the primary and secondary expected payer[16]

- If the primary or secondary expected payer indicates Medicare, then the payer category is assigned to Medicare. This categorization includes patients who are dually eligible for Medicare and Medicaid under Medicare.
- If not Medicare and the primary or secondary expected payer indicates Medicaid, then the payer category is Medicaid.
- If not Medicare or Medicaid and the primary or secondary expected payer indicates private insurance, then the payer category is private.
- If not Medicare, Medicaid, or private and the primary expected payer indicates self-pay or no charge, then the payer category is uninsured.
- Stays for other types of payers are not reported in this Statistical Brief because this is a mixed payer group and small numbers.

For this Statistical Brief, categorization of readmission counts and costs by expected payer was based on the index stay. The concordance between the expected payer coded at the index stay and the expected payer coded at readmission varies by payer: 98 percent for Medicare, 95 percent for Medicaid, 93 percent for private, and 80 percent for uninsured (percentages based on the 2013 NRD).

About HCUP

The Healthcare Cost and Utilization Project (HCUP, pronounced "H-Cup") is a family of health care databases and related software tools and products developed through a Federal-State-Industry partnership and sponsored by the Agency for Healthcare Research and Quality (AHRQ). HCUP databases bring together the data collection efforts of State data organizations, hospital associations, and private data organizations (HCUP Partners), and the Federal government to create a national information resource of encounter-level health care data. HCUP includes the largest collection of longitudinal hospital care data in the United States, with all-payer, encounter-level information beginning in 1988. These databases enable research on a broad range of health policy issues, including cost and quality of health services, medical practice patterns, access to health care programs, and outcomes of treatments at the national, State, and local market levels.

HCUP would not be possible without the contributions of the following data collection Partners from across the United States:

Alaska State Hospital and Nursing Home Association
Arizona Department of Health Services
Arkansas Department of Health
California Office of Statewide Health Planning and Development
Colorado Hospital Association
Connecticut Hospital Association
District of Columbia Hospital Association
Florida Agency for Health Care Administration
Georgia Hospital Association
Hawaii Health Information Corporation
Illinois Department of Public Health
Indiana Hospital Association
Iowa Hospital Association

Kansas Hospital Association
Kentucky Cabinet for Health and Family Services
Louisiana Department of Health and Hospitals
Maine Health Data Organization
Maryland Health Services Cost Review Commission
Massachusetts Center for Health Information and Analysis
Michigan Health & Hospital Association
Minnesota Hospital Association
Mississippi Department of Health
Missouri Hospital Industry Data Institute
Montana MHA - An Association of Montana Health Care Providers
Nebraska Hospital Association
Nevada Department of Health and Human Services
New Hampshire Department of Health & Human Services
New Jersey Department of Health
New Mexico Department of Health
New York State Department of Health
North Carolina Department of Health and Human Services
North Dakota (data provided by the Minnesota Hospital Association)
Ohio Hospital Association
Oklahoma State Department of Health
Oregon Association of Hospitals and Health Systems
Oregon Office of Health Analytics
Pennsylvania Health Care Cost Containment Council
Rhode Island Department of Health
South Carolina Budget & Control Board
South Dakota Association of Healthcare Organizations
Tennessee Hospital Association
Texas Department of State Health Services
Utah Department of Health
Vermont Association of Hospitals and Health Systems
Virginia Health Information
Washington State Department of Health
West Virginia Health Care Authority
Wisconsin Department of Health Services
Wyoming Hospital Association

About Statistical Briefs

HCUP Statistical Briefs are descriptive summary reports presenting statistics on hospital inpatient and emergency department use and costs, quality of care, access to care, medical conditions, procedures, patient populations, and other topics. The reports use HCUP administrative health care data.

About the NRD

The HCUP Nationwide Readmissions Database (NRD) is a calendar-year, discharge-level database constructed from the HCUP State Inpatient Databases (SID) with verified patient linkage numbers that can be used to track a person across hospitals within a State. The 2013 NRD is available for purchase through the HCUP Central Distributor. The NRD is designed to support various types of analyses of national readmission rates. The database includes discharges for patients with and without repeat hospital visits in a year and those who have died in the hospital. Repeat stays may or may not be related. The criteria to determine the relationship between hospital admissions is left to the analyst using the NRD. The NRD was constructed as a sample of convenience consisting of 100 percent of the eligible discharges. Discharge weights for national estimates are developed using the target universe of community hospitals (excluding rehabilitation and long-term acute care hospitals) in the United States. Over time, the sampling frame for the NRD will change; thus, the number of States contributing to the NRD will vary from year to year. The NRD is intended for national estimates only; no regional, State-, or hospital-specific estimates can be produced.

About the SID

The HCUP State Inpatient Databases (SID) are hospital inpatient databases from data organizations participating in HCUP. The SID contain the universe of the inpatient discharge abstracts in the participating HCUP States, translated into a uniform format to facilitate multistate comparisons and analyses. Together, the SID encompass more than 95 percent of all U.S. community hospital discharges. The SID can be used to investigate questions unique to one State, to compare data from two or more States, to conduct market-area variation analyses, and to identify State-specific trends in inpatient care utilization, access, charges, and outcomes.

About HCUPnet

HCUPnet is an online query system that offers instant access to the largest set of all-payer health care databases that are publicly available. HCUPnet has an easy step-by-step query system that creates tables and graphs of national and regional statistics as well as data trends for community hospitals in the United States. HCUPnet generates statistics using data from HCUP's National (Nationwide) Inpatient Sample (NIS), the Kids' Inpatient Database (KID), the Nationwide Emergency Department Sample (NEDS), the Nationwide Readmissions Database (NRD), the State Inpatient Databases (SID), and the State Emergency Department Databases (SEDD).

For More Information

For more information about HCUP, visit http://www.hcup-us.ahrq.gov/.

For additional HCUP statistics, visit HCUPnet, our interactive query system, at http://hcupnet.ahrq.gov/.

For information on other hospitalizations in the United States, refer to the following HCUP Statistical Briefs located at http://www.hcup-us.ahrq.gov/reports/statbriefs/statbriefs.jsp:

- Statistical Brief #180, Overview of Hospital Stays in the United States, 2012.
- Statistical Brief #181, Costs for Hospital Stays in the United States, 2012.
- Statistical Brief #186, Most Frequent Operating Room Procedures Performed in U.S. Hospitals, 2003–2012.
- Statistical Brief #162, Most Frequent Conditions in U.S. Hospitals, 2011.

End Notes

[1] Hines AL, Barrett ML, Jiang HJ, Steiner CA. Conditions With the Largest Number of Adult Hospital Readmissions by Payer, 2011. HCUP Statistical Brief #172. April 2014. Agency for Healthcare Research and Quality, Rockville, MD. http://www.hcupus.ahrq.gov/reports/statbriefs/sb172-Conditions-Readmissions-Payer.pdf. Accessed October 22, 2015.

[2] Minott J. Reducing Hospital Readmissions. Washington, DC: Academy Health; November 2008. http://www.academyhealth.org/files/publications/ReducingHospitalReadmissions.pdf Accessed June 12, 2015.

[3] Ibid.

[4] Ibid.

[5] Boccuti C, Casillas G. Aiming for Fewer Hospital U-turns: The Medicare Hospital Readmissions Reduction Program. Menlo Park, CA: The Henry J. Kaiser Family Foundation; January 2015. http://kff.org/medicare/issue-brief/aiming-for-fewerhospital-u-turns-the-medicare-hospital-readmission-reduction-program/. Accessed June 12, 2015.

[6] Boccuti C, Casillas G. Aiming for Fewer Hospital U-turns: The Medicare Hospital Readmissions Reduction Program. Menlo Park, CA: The Henry J. Kaiser Family Foundation; January 2015. http://kff.org/medicare/issue-brief/aiming-for-fewer-hospital-u-turns-themedicare-hospital-readmission-reduction-program/. Accessed June 12, 2015.

[7] Thorpe JH, Cascio T. Medicare Hospital Readmissions Reduction Program. Legal Notes. 2011;3(4):1–4. http://www.rwjf.org/content/dam/farm/reports/issue briefs/2011/rwjf71483. Accessed June 12, 2015.

[8] Agency for Healthcare Research and Quality. HCUPnet Web site. http://hcupnet.ahrq.gov/. Accessed June 29, 2015.

[9] HCUP Clinical Classifications Software (CCS). Healthcare Cost and Utilization Project (HCUP). Healthcare Cost and Utilization Project. Rockville, MD: Agency for Healthcare Research and Quality. Updated November 2014. http://www.hcup-us.ahrq.gov/tools software/ccs/ccs.jsp. Accessed January 7, 2015.

[10] Centers for Medicare & Medicaid Services. Measure Methodology. https://www.cms.gov/Medicare/Quality-Initiatives-PatientAssessment-Instruments/HospitalQualityInits/Measure-Methodology.html. Accessed October 1, 2015.

[11] Boccuti C, Casillas G. Aiming for Fewer Hospital U-turns: The Medicare Hospital Readmissions Reduction Program. Menlo Park, CA: The Henry J. Kaiser Family Foundation; January 2015. http://kff.org/medicare/issue-brief/aiming-for-fewer-hospital-u-turns-themedicare-hospital-readmission-reduction-program/. Accessed October 1, 2015.

[12] Agency for Healthcare Research and Quality. HCUP Cost-to-Charge Ratio (CCR) Files. Healthcare Cost and Utilization Project (HCUP). 2001–2011. Rockville, MD: Agency for Healthcare Research and Quality, Rockville, MD. Updated December 2014. http://www.hcup-us.ahrq.gov/db/state/costtocharge.jsp. Accessed January 7, 2015.

[13] U.S. Bureau of Economic Analysis. National Income and Product Account Tables, Table 1.1.4 Price Indexes for Gross Domestic Product. http://www.bea.gov/iTable/iTable.cfm?ReqID=9&step=1#reqid=9&step=1&isuri=1. Accessed October 13, 2015.

[14] For additional information about the NHEA, see Centers for Medicare & Medicaid Services (CMS). National Health Expenditure Data. CMS Web site May 2014. http://www.cms.gov/Research-Statistics-Data-and-Systems/Statistics-Trends-and-Reports/NationalHealthExpendData/index.html?redirect=/NationalHealthExpendData/. Accessed January 7, 2015.

[15] American Hospital Association. TrendWatch Chartbook, 2014. Table 4.2. Distribution of Inpatient vs. Outpatient Revenues, 1992– 2012. http://www.aha.org/research/reports/tw/chartbook/2014/table4-2.pdf. Accessed January 7, 2015.

[16] The 2013 NRD available for purchase through the HCUP Central Distributor includes the data element for the primary expected payer but not the data element for the secondary expected payer.

In: Significant Health Statistics
Editor: Christopher Barrett

ISBN: 978-1-63484-563-2

Chapter 6

HOSPITALIZATIONS FOR PATIENTS AGED 85 AND OVER IN THE UNITED STATES, 2000–2010*

Shaleah Levant, MPH, Karishma Chari, MPH, and Carol J. DeFrances, PhD

KEY FINDINGS

Data from the National Hospital Discharge Survey

- In 2010, adults aged 85 and over accounted for only 2% of the U.S. population but 9% of hospital discharges.
- From 2000 through 2010, the rate of hospitalizations for adults aged 85 and over declined from 605 to 553 hospitalizations per 1,000 population, a 9% decrease.
- The rate of fractures and other injuries was higher for adults aged 85 and over (51 per 1,000 population) than for adults aged 65–74 (9 per 1,000 population) and 75–84 (23 per 1,000 population).
- Adults aged 85 and over were less likely than those aged 65–74 and 75–84 to be discharged home and more likely to die in the hospital.

---

* This is an edited, reformatted and augmented version of NCHS Data Brief No. 182, issued by the National Center for Health Statistics, January 2015.

From 2000 through 2010, the number of adults aged 85 and over in the United States rose 31%, from 4.2 million to 5.5 million, and in 2010, this age group represented almost 14% of the population aged 65 and over [1]. It is estimated that by 2050, more than 21% of adults over age 65 will be aged 85 and over [2]. Given this increase, adults aged 85 and over are likely to account for an increasing share of hospital utilization and costs in the coming years [3]. This report describes hospitalizations for adults aged 85 and over with comparisons to adults aged 65–74 and 75–84.

Keywords: inpatient care, health care utilization, National Hospital Discharge Survey

What Percentage of Hospital Care Was Provided to Adults Aged 85 and Over?

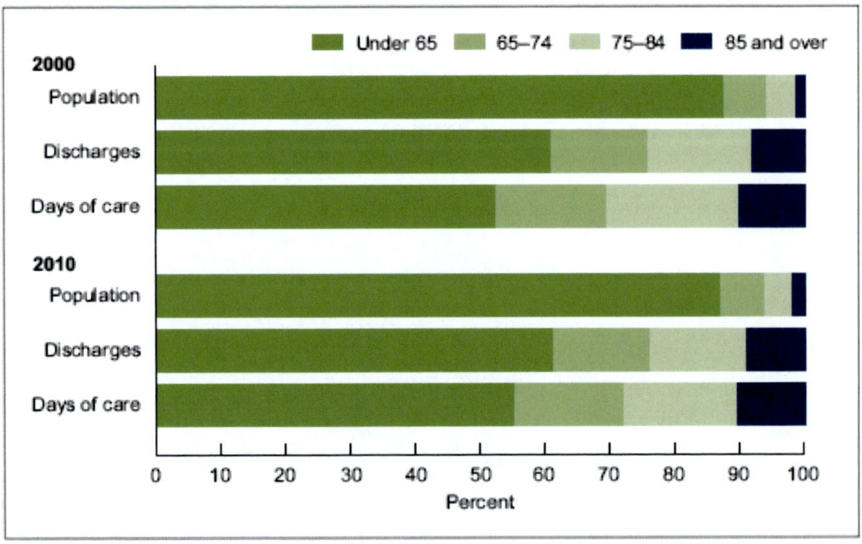

Source: CDC/NCHS, National Hospital Discharge Survey, 2000–2010.
Note: Population is the U.S. civilian noninstitutionalized population.

Figure 1. Population, discharges, and days of care, by age: United States, 2000 and 2010.

- In 2000, adults aged 85 and over accounted for only 2% of the U.S. population but 8% of hospital discharges. In 2010, adults aged 85 and over still accounted for 2% of the U.S. population but accounted for 9% of hospital discharges (Figure 1).

- In 2000 and 2010, adults aged 85 and over accounted for 12% and 14%, respectively, of those aged 65 and over. However, adults aged 85 and over accounted for more than 20% of hospital discharges for those aged 65 and over for both years.
- Adults aged 85 and over accounted for a disproportionate share of the total days of care, 10% in 2000 and 11% in 2010.

Were Adults Aged 85 and Over More Likely Than Other Age Groups to Be Hospitalized?

- The hospitalization rate for adults aged 85 and over declined by 9% from 2000 through 2010, from 605 to 553 per 1,000 population, respectively (Figure 2).
- From 2000 through 2010, the hospitalization rate for adults aged 85 and over remained significantly higher than the rates for adults under age 65, aged 65–74, and aged 75–84.
- In 2010, the hospitalization rate for adults aged 85 and over (553 per 1,000 population) was more than five times higher than the rate for adults under 65 (80 per 1,000 population).

What Were Common Causes of Hospitalization for Adults Aged 85 and Over?

- In 2010, congestive heart failure (43 per 1,000 population) was the most frequent first-listed diagnosis for adults aged 85 and over, but in 2000 and 2005, pneumonia (51 and 52 per 1,000 population, respectively) was the most common first-listed diagnosis for adults aged 85 and over (Table).
- Hospitalization rates for congestive heart failure, pneumonia, stroke, and hip fracture decreased from 2000 through 2010 for adults aged 85 and over, and the rates for urinary tract infections and septicemia increased from 2000 through 2010.

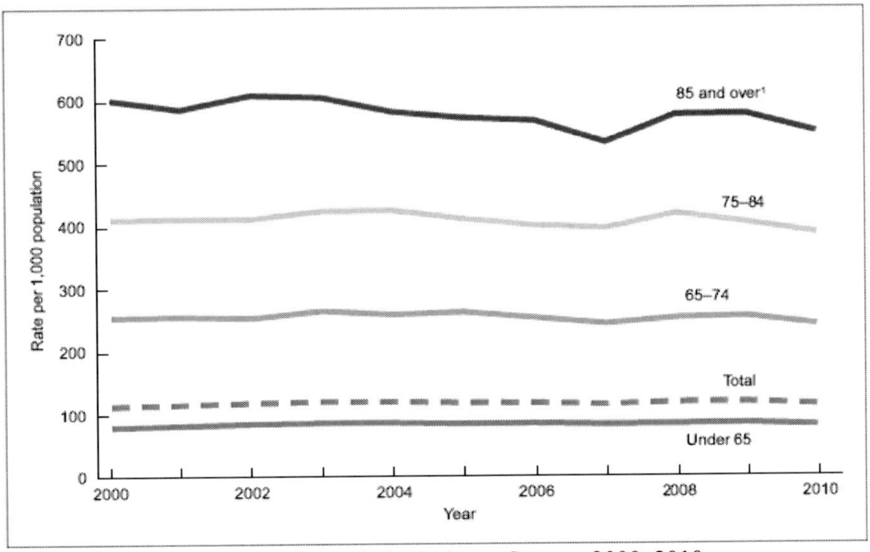

Source: CDC/NCHS, National Hospital Discharge Survey, 2000–2010.

[1] Rate of hospitalization exceeds the rate for younger age groups for every year from 2000 through 2010 ($p < 0.05$).

Figure 2. Hospitalizations, by age: United States, 2000–2010.

Table. Common causes of hospitalization for adults aged 85 and over: United States, 2010

First-listed diagnosis	2000	2005	2010	Percent change[1] (2000 to 2010)
		Rate of hospitalization per 1,000 population		
Congestive heart failure	48	47	43	–9.5
Pneumonia	51	52	34	–32.8
Urinary tract infection	19	24	30	+55.9
Septicemia	15	18	28	+84.8
Stroke	37	27	28	–25.0
Hip fracture	28	23	21	–25.4

Source: CDC/NCHS, National Hospital Discharge Survey, 2000–2010.

Note: First-listed diagnosis is considered to be the main cause or reason for the hospitalization. The diagnoses were chosen because they were the top six first-listed diagnoses in 2010.

[1] Percent change for each diagnosis is significant from 2000 through 2010 ($p < 0.05$).

How Likely Were Adults Aged 85 and Over to Be Hospitalized for Injury?

- The rate of all injuries for adults aged 85 and over (51 per 1,000 population) was higher than the rates for adults aged 65–74 and 75–84 (9 and 23 per 1,000 population, respectively) (Figure 3).
- The rate of hip fractures for adults aged 85 and over (21 per 1,000 population) was higher than the rates for adults aged 65–74 and 75–84 (2 and 8 per 1,000 population, respectively).
- The rate of other fractures for adults aged 85 and over (18 per 1,000 population) was higher than the rates for adults aged 65–74 and 75–84 (4 and 10 per 1,000 population, respectively).
- The rate of other injuries for adults aged 85 and over (12 per 1,000 population) was higher than the rates for adults aged 65–74 and 75–84 (3 and 6 per 1,000 population, respectively).

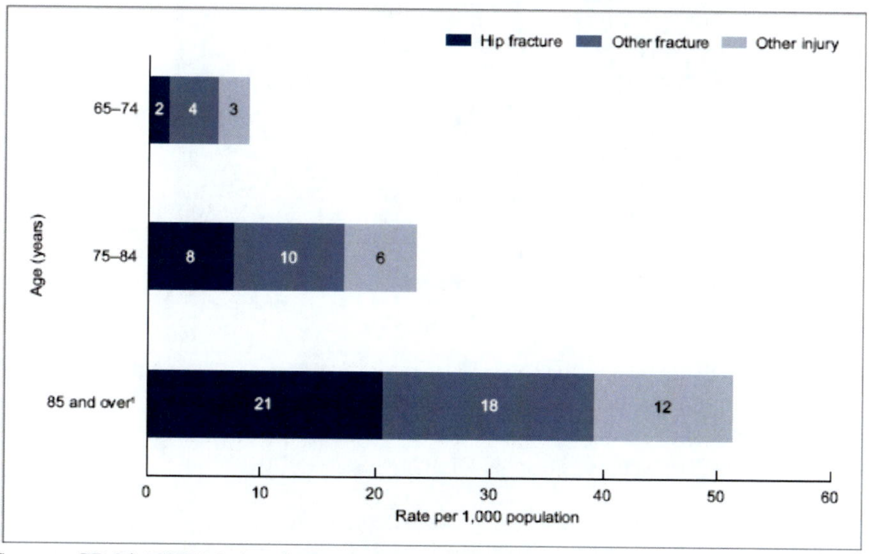

Source: CDC/NCHS National Hospital Discharge Survey, 2010.

[1] All differences between adults aged 85 and over and both the 65–74 and the 75–84 age groups are statistically significant ($p < 0.05$).

Figure 3. Injury hospitalizations, by age and selected diagnoses: United States, 2010.

Where Were Adults Aged 85 and Over Discharged to After Hospitalization?

- Adults aged 85 and over were less likely to be discharged to their homes (44%) than adults aged 65–74 and 75–84 (71% and 58%, respectively), and they were more likely to be discharged to a long-term care facility (36% compared with 14% and 24%, respectively) (Figure 4).
- Adults aged 85 and over were more likely to die during hospitalization than those aged 65–74 and 75–84 (6% compared with 3% and 4%, respectively).

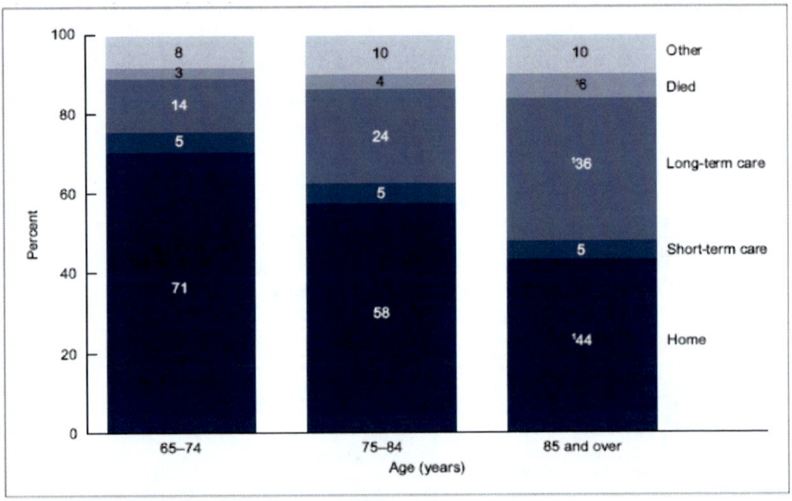

[1]Differences between adults aged 85 and over and both the 65–74 and the 75–84 age groups are statistically significant ($p < 0.05$).
Note: Percentages may not add to totals due to rounding.
Source: CDC/NCHS National Hospital Discharge Survey, 2010.

Figure 4. Discharge status, by age group: United States, 2010.

Summary

This analysis examined hospitalizations for adults aged 85 and over from 2000 through 2010 and compared these adults with adults aged 65–74 and 75–84. In 2010, adults aged 85 and over accounted for 2% of the total U.S.

population. However, they accounted for a disproportionate share of hospital discharges and days of care—9% and 11%, respectively. The hospitalization rate for adults aged 85 and over decreased between 2000 and 2010, but it remained significantly higher than all other age groups.

The life expectancy of people who reach age 85 is another 6.5 years; those who reach age 90 can expect to live another 4.6 years [4]. As the number of adults aged 85 and over in the United States continues to rise, the recognition of age differences in the utilization and provision of inpatient services among this population will be important. Prevention efforts to keep adults aged 85 and over out of inpatient settings will help reduce health care costs and maintain quality of life. For example, falling causes more than 95% of hip fractures, one of the leading causes of hospital admission, and can ultimately result in nursing home admission, long-term functional impairment, and increased mortality [5].

DEFINITIONS

First-listed diagnosis: The principal diagnosis, considered to be the main cause or reason for the hospitalization. Diagnoses are coded according to the *International Classification of Diseases, Ninth Revision, Clinical Modification* (ICD–9–CM) coding system [6]. The ICD–9–CM codes for the first-listed diagnoses included in this report are the following:

Congestive heart failure—codes 428.0 and 428.2–428.4
Pneumonia—codes 480–486
Stroke—codes 430–438
Urinary tract infection—code 599.0
Hip fracture—code 820
Other fracture—codes 800–819 and 821–829
Other injury—codes 830–959

Rate: The number of hospitalizations per unit of population (e.g., per 10,000 population). Using rates removes the influence of different population sizes (e.g., for adults aged 75–84 and 85 and over in the same year or for the same age group over multiple years) so that data can be compared across these groups. For 2000–2010, rates were calculated using U.S. Census Bureau 2000-based postcensal civilian population estimates.

DATA SOURCE AND METHODS

Data for this report are from the National Hospital Discharge Survey (NHDS), a national probability sample survey of discharges from nonfederal, short-stay hospitals or general hospitals in the United States. The survey was conducted annually until 2010 by the Centers for Disease Control and Prevention's (CDC) National Center for Health Statistics, Division of Health Care Statistics. NHDS uses a modified three-stage design. Units selected at the first stage consist of either hospitals or geographic areas, such as counties, groups of counties, or metropolitan statistical areas. Within a sampled geographic area, hospitals are selected. Finally at the last stage, systematic random sampling is used to select discharges within sampled hospitals. Survey data on hospital discharges were obtained from the hospitals' administrative data. Note that if an individual is admitted to the hospital multiple times during the survey year, that individual could be counted more than once in NHDS.

Because of the complex multistage design of NHDS, the survey data must be inflated or weighted to produce national estimates. Estimates of inpatient care presented in this report exclude newborns. More details about the design of NHDS have been published elsewhere [7].

A weighted least-squares regression method [8], based on all 11 years of NHDS data from 2000 through 2010, was used to test for linear trends in the table and all figures. This is the case even if only selected years of data are shown. A p value of less 0.05 indicated statistical significance. Differences among subgroups were evaluated with two-tailed t tests using $p < 0.05$ as the level of significance. Terms that express differences such as "higher," "lower," "largest," "smallest," "leading," "increased," or "decreased," were used only when the differences were statistically significant. When a comparison is described as "similar," it means no statistically significant difference was found. All comparisons reported in the text were statistically significant unless otherwise indicated. Data analyses were performed using the statistical packages SAS version 9.3 (SAS Institute, Cary, N.C.) and SUDAAN version 11.0 (RTI International, Research Triangle Park, N.C.).

ABOUT THE AUTHORS

Shaleah Levant, Karishma Chari, and Carol J. DeFrances are with CDC's National Center for Health Statistics, Division of Health Care Statistics.

REFERENCES

[1] Werner CA. The older population: 2010. C2010BR–09. U.S. Census Bureau: Washington, DC. 2011.

[2] Vincent GK, Velkoff VA. The next four decades. The older population in the United States: 2010 to 2050. Current population reports P25–1138. U.S. Census Bureau: Washington, DC. 2010.

[3] Federal Interagency Forum on Aging-Related Statistics. Older Americans 2012: Key indicators of well-being. Federal Interagency Forum on Aging-Related Statistics. Washington, DC: U.S. Government Printing Office. 2012.

[4] Murphy SL, Xu JQ, Kochanek KD. Deaths: Preliminary data for 2010. National vital statistics reports; vol 60 no 4. Hyattsville, MD: National Center for Health Statistics. 2012. Available from: http://www.cdc.gov/nchs/data/nvsr/nvsr60/nvsr60_04.pdf.

[5] National Center for Injury Prevention and Control. Home and recreational safety: Hip fractures among older adults. 2013. Available from: http://www.cdc.gov/homeandrecreationalsafety/falls/adulthipfx.html.

[6] CDC. International classification of diseases, ninth revision, clinical modification. 6th ed. 2006. Available from: http://www.cdc.gov/nchs/icd/icd9cm.htm.

[7] Hall MJ, DeFrances CJ, Williams SN, et al. National Hospital Discharge Survey: 2007 summary. National health statistics reports; no 29. Hyattsville, MD: National Center for Health Statistics. 2010. Available from: http://www.cdc.gov/nchs/data/nhsr/nhsr029.pdf.

[8] Gillum BS, Graves EJ, Kozak LJ. Trends in hospital utilization: United States, 1988–92. National Center for Health Statistics. Vital Health Stat 13(124). 1996. Available from: http://www.cdc.gov/nchs/data/series/sr_13/sr13_124.pdf.

In: Significant Health Statistics
Editor: Christopher Barrett
ISBN: 978-1-63484-563-2

Chapter 7

PREVALENCE OF OBESITY AMONG ADULTS AND YOUTH: UNITED STATES, 2011–2014*

Cynthia L. Ogden, PhD, Margaret D. Carroll, MSPH, Cheryl D. Fryar, MSPH, and Katherine M. Flegal, PhD

KEY FINDINGS

Data from the National Health and Nutrition Examination Survey

- In 2011–2014, the prevalence of obesity was just over 36% in adults and 17% in youth.
- The prevalence of obesity was higher in women (38.3%) than in men (34.3%). Among all youth, no difference was seen by sex.
- The prevalence of obesity was higher among middle-aged (40.2%) and older (37.0%) adults than younger (32.3%) adults.
- The prevalence of obesity was higher among non-Hispanic white, non-Hispanic black, and Hispanic adults and youth than among non-Hispanic Asian adults and youth.

---

* This is an edited, reformatted and augmented version of NCHS Data Brief No. 219, issued by the National Center for Health Statistics, November 2015.

- From 1999 through 2014, obesity prevalence increased among adults and youth. However, among youth, prevalence did not change from 2003–2004 through 2013–2014.

Obesity is associated with health risks [1, 2]. Monitoring the prevalence of obesity is relevant for public health programs that focus on reducing or preventing obesity. No significant changes were seen in either adult or childhood obesity prevalence in the United States between 2003–2004 and 2011–2012 [3]. This report provides the most recent national data on obesity prevalence by sex, age, and race and Hispanic origin, using data for 2011–2014. Overall prevalence estimates from 1999–2000 through 2013–2014 are also presented.

Keyword: National Health and Nutrition Examination Survey

What Was the Prevalence of Obesity Among Adults in 2011–2014?

The prevalence of obesity was 36.5% (crude estimate) among U.S. adults during 2011–2014. Overall, the prevalence of obesity among middle-aged adults aged 40–59 (40.2%) and older adults aged 60 and over (37.0%) was higher than among younger adults aged 20–39 (32.3%). No significant difference in prevalence was observed between middle-aged and older adults (Figure 1).

Overall, the prevalence of obesity among women (38.3%) was higher than among men (34.3%). For adults aged 20–39 and 40–59, the prevalence of obesity was higher among women than among men, but the difference between older women and men aged 60 and over was not significant.

Among both men and women, the prevalence of obesity followed a similar pattern by age. Men aged 40–59 (38.3%) had a higher prevalence of obesity than men aged 20–39 (30.3%). Women aged 40–59 (42.1%) had a higher prevalence of obesity than women aged 20–39 (34.4%). The prevalence of obesity among men and women aged 20–39 was lower than among men and women aged 60 and over, except the difference for men was not significant.

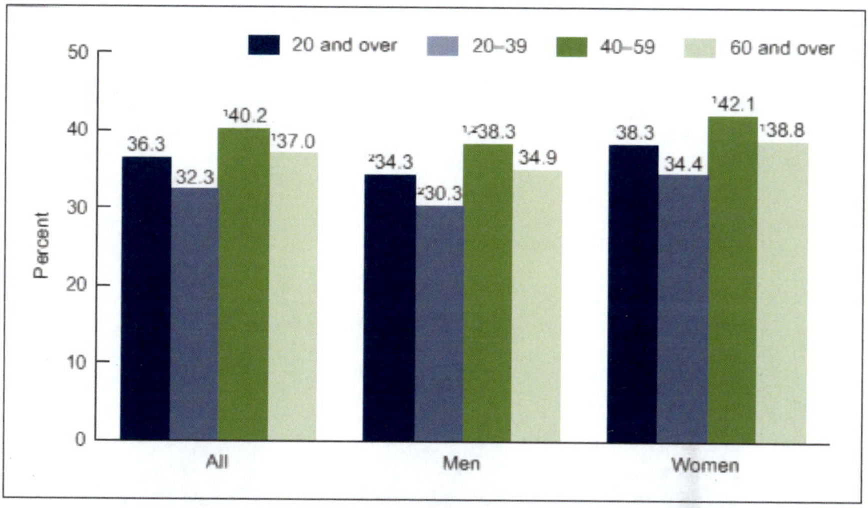

Source: CDC/NCHS, National Health and Nutrition Examination Survey, 2011–2014.

Notes: Totals were age-adjusted by the direct method to the 2000 U.S. census population using the age groups 20–39, 40–59, and 60 and over. Crude estimates are 36.5% for all, 34.5% for men, and 38.5% for women.

[1]Significantly different from those aged 20–39.

[2]Significantly different from women of the same age group.

Figure 1. Prevalence of obesity among adults aged 20 and over, by sex and age: United States, 2011–2014.

WERE THERE DIFFERENCES IN THE PREVALENCE OF OBESITY AMONG ADULTS BY RACE AND HISPANIC ORIGIN IN 2011–2014?

The prevalence of obesity was lowest among non-Hispanic Asian adults (11.7%), followed by non-Hispanic white (34.5%), Hispanic (42.5%), and non-Hispanic black (48.1%) adults. All differences were significant. The pattern among women was similar to the pattern in the overall adult population. The prevalence of obesity was 11.9% in non-Hispanic Asian, 35.5% in non-Hispanic white, 45.7% in Hispanic, and 56.9% in non-Hispanic black women. The prevalence of obesity was lower in non-Hispanic Asian (11.2%) men compared with non-Hispanic white (33.6%), non-Hispanic black (37.5%), and Hispanic (39.0%) men. No difference in obesity prevalence was observed between non-Hispanic black and non-Hispanic white men, nor was there a difference between non-Hispanic black and Hispanic men (Figure 2).

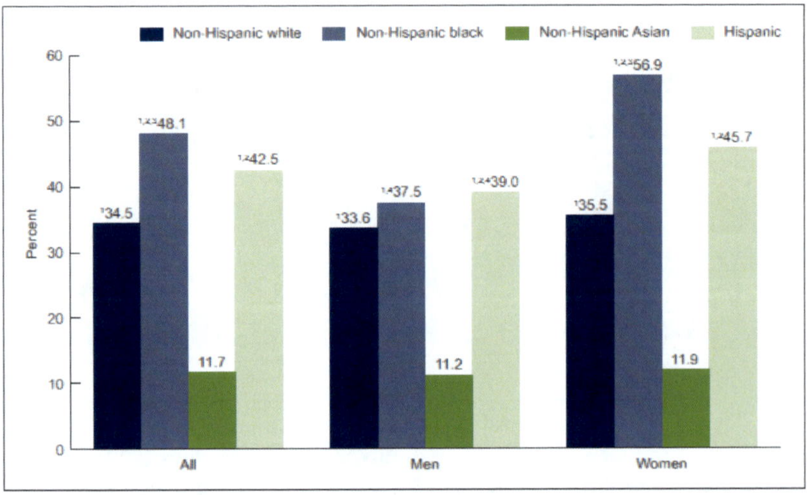

Source: CDC/NCHS, National Health and Nutrition Examination Survey, 2011–2014.
[1]Significantly different from non-Hispanic Asian persons.
[2]Significantly different from non-Hispanic white persons.
[3]Significantly different from Hispanic persons.
[4]Significantly different from women of the same race and Hispanic origin.
Note: All estimates are age-adjusted by the direct method to the 2000 U.S. census population using the age groups 20–39, 40–59, and 60 and over.

Figure 2. Prevalence of obesity among adults aged 20 and over, by sex and race and Hispanic origin: United States, 2011–2014.

The only differences by sex were found among non-Hispanic black and Hispanic adults. The prevalence of obesity among non-Hispanic black women was 56.9% compared with 37.5% in non-Hispanic black men. The prevalence of obesity was 45.7% among Hispanic women compared with 39.0% in Hispanic men.

What Was the Prevalence of Obesity Among Youth Aged 2–19 Years in 2011–2014?

The prevalence of obesity among U.S. youth was 17.0% in 2011–2014. Overall, the prevalence of obesity among preschool-aged children (2–5 years)

(8.9%) was lower than among school-aged children (6–11 years) (17.5%) and adolescents (12–19 years) (20.5%). The same pattern was seen in both males and females (Figure 3).

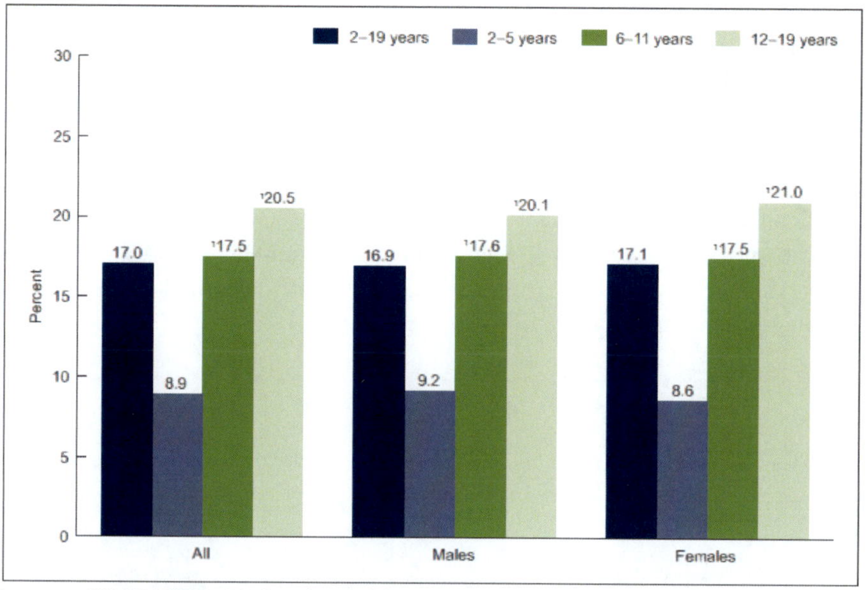

Source: CDC/NCHS, National Health and Nutrition Examination Survey, 2011–2014[1]Significantly different from those aged 2–5 years.

Figure 3. Prevalence of obesity among youth aged 2–19 years, by sex and age: United States, 2011–2014.

Were There Differences in the Prevalence of Obesity Among Youth Aged 2–19 Years by Race and Hispanic Origin in 2011–2014?

The prevalence of obesity among non-Hispanic Asian youth (8.6%) was lower than among non-Hispanic white (14.7%), non-Hispanic black (19.5%), and Hispanic (21.9%) youth. The prevalence of obesity among non-Hispanic white youth was lower than in non-Hispanic black and Hispanic youth, but no significant difference was observed between non-Hispanic black and Hispanic youth.

The pattern among females was similar to the pattern in the overall population, except the prevalence was not significantly different in non-Hispanic white females compared with non-Hispanic black females. The prevalence of obesity was 5.3% in non-Hispanic Asian, 15.1% in non-Hispanic white, 20.7% in non-Hispanic black, and 21.4% in Hispanic females.

Among males, the prevalence of obesity was lower in non-Hispanic Asian (11.8%) males compared with non-Hispanic black (18.4%) and Hispanic (22.4%) males, but no significant difference was seen between non-Hispanic Asian (11.8%) and non-Hispanic white (14.3%) males. Differences between non-Hispanic white, non-Hispanic black, and Hispanic males were statistically significant (Figure 4).

The only difference by sex was found among non-Hispanic Asian youth—the prevalence was 11.8% in non-Hispanic Asian males and 5.3% in non-Hispanic Asian females.

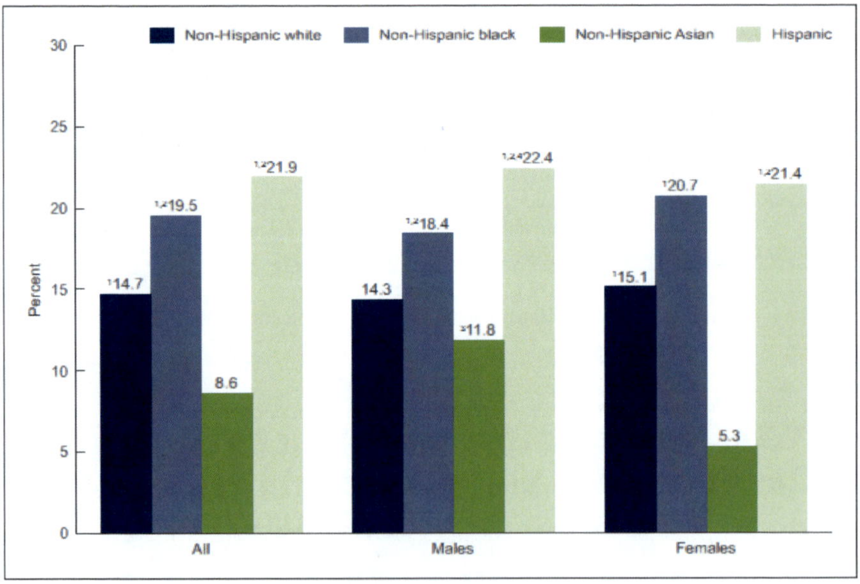

[1]Significantly different from non-Hispanic Asian persons.
[2]Significantly different from non-Hispanic white persons.
[3]Significantly different from females of the same race and Hispanic origin.
[4]Significantly different from non-Hispanic black persons.
Source: CDC/NCHS, National Health and Nutrition Examination Survey, 2011–2014.

Figure 4. Prevalence of obesity among youth aged 2–19 years, by sex and race and Hispanic origin: United States, 2011–2014.

WHAT ARE THE TRENDS IN ADULT AND CHILDHOOD OBESITY?

From 1999–2000 through 2013–2014, a significant increase in obesity was observed in both adults and youth. Between 2003–2004 and 2013–2014, however, no change in prevalence was seen among youth. No change in obesity prevalence among youth was noted between 2011–2012 and 2013–2014, and the observed change in adults between 2011–2012 and 2013–2014 was not significant (Figure 5).

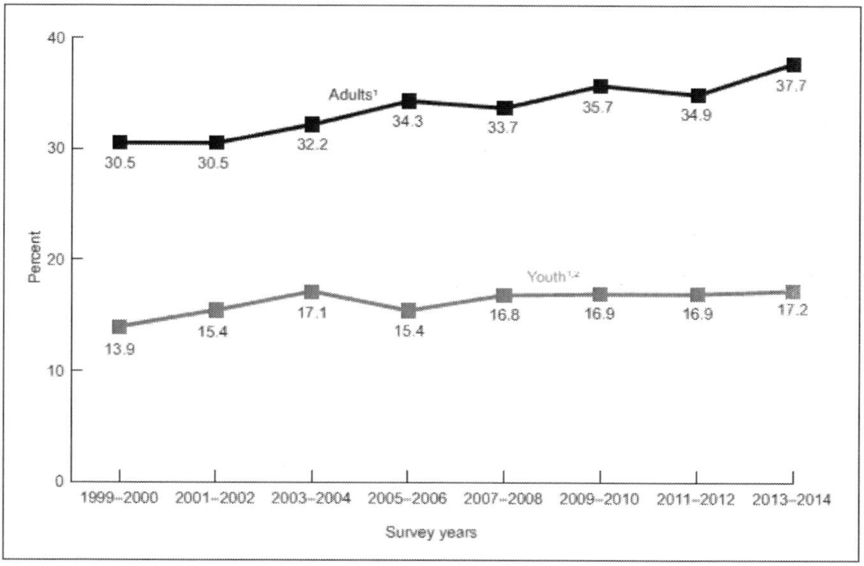

[1]Significant increasing linear trend from 1999–2000 through 2013–2014.
[2]Test for linear trend for 2003–2004 through 2013–2014 not significant ($p > 0.05$).
Note: All adult estimates are age-adjusted by the direct method to the 2000 U.S. census population using the age groups 20–39, 40–59, and 60 and over.
Source: CDC/NCHS, National Health and Nutrition Examination Survey.

Figure 5. Trends in obesity prevalence among adults aged 20 and over (age-adjusted) and youth aged 2–19 years: United States, 1999–2000 through 2013–2014.

SUMMARY

More than one-third of adults and 17% of youth in the United States were obese in 2011–2014. The prevalence of obesity was higher among women than among men overall and higher among non-Hispanic black and Hispanic adults compared with other racial and Hispanic origin groups. Among youth, no difference in obesity prevalence was seen between males and females, except among non-Hispanic Asian youth.

Obesity prevalence was lower among non-Hispanic Asian adults compared with other racial and Hispanic origin groups. No difference in obesity prevalence was observed between non-Hispanic black and Hispanic men. However, the prevalence was higher among non-Hispanic black women compared with Hispanic women. Among youth, the prevalence of obesity was lowest among non-Hispanic Asian youth, but no significant difference in prevalence was seen between non-Hispanic white and non-Hispanic Asian males. Among males, the prevalence of obesity was lower among non-Hispanic black compared with Hispanic youth. However, among females, no difference in prevalence was observed between non-Hispanic black and Hispanic youth.

Trends in obesity prevalence show no increase among youth since 2003–2004, but trends do show increases in both adults and youth from 1999–2000 through 2013–2014. No significant differences between 2011–2012 and 2013–2014 were seen in either youth or adults.

Obesity is defined using cut points of body mass index (BMI). BMI does not measure body fat directly, and the relationship between BMI and body fat varies by sex, age, and race and Hispanic origin [4, 5]. Morbidity and mortality risk may vary between different racial and Hispanic origin groups at the same BMI. Some studies suggest that among some Asian subgroups, health and mortality risks may begin at a lower BMI compared with other racial and Hispanic origin groups [6–8].

The definition of obesity is based on BMI for both youth and adults, but the definitions are not directly comparable. Among adults, there is a set cut point based on health risk, while among children the definition is statistical and is based on a comparison to a reference population [9].

The prevalence of obesity among U.S. adults remains higher than the Healthy People 2020 goal of 30.5% [10]. Although the overall prevalence of childhood obesity is higher than the Healthy People 2020 goal of 14.5%, the prevalence of obesity among children aged 2–5 years is below the goal of 9.4%.

Definitions

Non-Hispanic Asian: Primarily comprises persons of Chinese, Asian Indian, Korean, Filipino, Vietnamese, and Japanese descent.

Obesity: BMI was calculated as weight in kilograms divided by height in meters squared, rounded to one decimal place. Obesity in adults was defined as a BMI of greater than or equal to 30. Obesity in youth was defined as a BMI of greater than or equal to the age- and sex-specific 95th percentile of the 2000 CDC growth charts [9].

Data Source and Methods

Data from the National Health and Nutrition Examination Surveys (NHANES) for survey years 1999–2000, 2001–2002, 2003–2004, 2005–2006, 2007–2008, 2009–2010, 2011–2012, and 2013–2014 were used for these analyses. Data from NHANES 2011–2014 (4 years of data) were used to test differences between demographic subgroups, thus increasing the sample size and the ability to detect a difference in the prevalence. In testing for trends in obesity, eight 2-year cycles were used: 1999–2000, 2001–2002, 2003–2004, 2005–2006, 2007–2008, 2009–2010, 2011–2012, and 2013–2014. Because previous research found no increase in obesity prevalence from 2003– 2004 through 2011–2012 [3], analyses of linear trends were also conducted between 2003–2004 and 2013–2014.

NHANES is a cross-sectional survey designed to monitor the health and nutritional status of the civilian noninstitutionalized U.S. population [11]. The survey consists of interviews conducted in participants' homes and standardized physical examinations conducted in mobile examination centers.

The NHANES sample is selected through a complex, multistage probability design. In 2011–2012 and 2013–2014, non-Hispanic black, non-Hispanic Asian, and Hispanic persons, among other groups, were oversampled to obtain reliable estimates for these population subgroups. Race- and Hispanic origin-specific estimates reflect individuals reporting only one race; those reporting more than one race are included in the total but are not reported separately.

Examination sample weights, which account for the differential probabilities of selection, nonresponse, and noncoverage, were incorporated into the estimation process. All variance estimates accounted for the complex survey design by using Taylor series linearization. Pregnant females were excluded from analyses.

Prevalence estimates for the adult population aged 20 and over were age-adjusted using the direct method to the 2000 U.S. census population using the age groups 20–39, 40–59, and 60 and over. Differences between groups were tested using a univariate t statistic at the $p < 0.05$ significance level. All differences reported are statistically significant unless otherwise indicated. Adjustments were not made for multiple comparisons. Statistical analyses were conducted using the SAS System for Windows, release 9.3 (SAS Institute Inc., Cary, N.C.) and SUDAAN, release 11.1 (RTI International, Research Triangle Park, N.C.).

About the Authors

Cynthia L. Ogden, Margaret D. Carroll, Cheryl D. Fryar, and Katherine M. Flegal are with CDC's National Center for Health Statistics, Division of Health and Nutrition Examination Surveys.

References

[1] Clinical guidelines on the identification, evaluation, and treatment of overweight and obesity in adults—The evidence report. *Obes. Res.* 6 Suppl 2:51S–209S. 1998.

[2] U.S. Department of Health and Human Services, Office of the Surgeon General. The surgeon general's vision for a healthy and fit nation. Rockville, MD: 2010.

[3] Ogden CL, Carroll MD, Kit BK, Flegal KM. Prevalence of childhood and adult obesity in the United States, 2011–2012. *JAMA* 311(8):806–14. 2014.

[4] Flegal KM, Ogden CL, Yanovski JA, Freedman DS, Shepherd JA, Graubard BI, Borrud LG. High adiposity and high body mass index-for-age in US children and adolescents overall and by race-ethnic group. *Am. J. Clin. Nutr.* 91(4):1020–6. 2010.

[5] Deurenberg P, Deurenberg-Yap M, Guricci S. Asians are different from Caucasians and from each other in their body mass index/body fat per cent relationship. *Obes. Rev.* 3(3):141–6. 2002.

[6] Nguyen TT, Adair LS, Suchindran CM, He K, Popkin BM. The association between body mass index and hypertension is different between East and Southeast Asians. *Am. J. Clin. Nutr.* 89(6):1905–12. 2009.

[7] Jafar TH, Islam M, Poulter N, Hatcher J, Schmid CH, Levey AS, Chaturvedi N. Children in South Asia have higher body mass-adjusted blood pressure levels than white children in the United States: A comparative study. *Circulation* 111(10):1291–7. 2005.

[8] Zheng W, McLerran DF, Rolland B, Zhang X, Inoue M, Matsuo K, et al. Association between body-mass index and risk of death in more than 1 million Asians. *N. Engl. J. Med.* 364(8):719–29. 2011.

[9] Ogden CL, Flegal KM. Changes in terminology for childhood overweight and obesity. National health statistics reports; no 25. Hyattsville, MD: *National Center for Health Statistics*. 2010.

[10] U.S. Department of Health and Human Services, Office of Disease Prevention and Health Promotion. Healthy People 2020 topics and objectives: Nutrition and weight status. Washington, DC. Available from: http://www.healthypeople.gov/2020/topics-objectives/topic/nutriation-andweight-status?topicid=29.

[11] Johnson CL, Dohrmann SM, Burt VL, Mohadjer LK. National Health and Nutrition Examination Survey: Sample design, 2011–2014. National Center for Health Statistics. Vital Health Stat 2(162). 2014.

In: Significant Health Statistics
Editor: Christopher Barrett
ISBN: 978-1-63484-563-2

Chapter 8

PREVALENCE OF OBESITY AMONG CHILDREN AND ADOLESCENTS IN THE UNITED STATES AND CANADA*

Margaret D. Carroll, MSPH, Tanya Navaneelan, MSc, Shirley Bryan, PhD, and Cynthia L. Ogden, PhD

KEY FINDINGS

- In the late 1970s, the prevalence of childhood obesity was the same in Canada and the United States, but recently the prevalence is 4.5 percentage points higher in the United States than in Canada.
- No change has been seen over the last decade in the prevalence of obesity among children and adolescents in Canada or the United States.
- The prevalence of obesity among children and adolescents aged 3–19 in Canada was lower (13.0%) than in the United States (17.5%) in recent years.
- There was no difference between Canada and the United States in the prevalence of obesity among children aged 3–6 years.

---

* This is an edited, reformatted and augmented version of NCHS Data Brief No. 211, issued by the National Center for Health Statistics, August 2015.

- In the non-Hispanic white population, the prevalence of obesity among girls was lower in Canada than in the United States, but there was no difference between the two countries among boys.

About one-quarter of Canadian adults and more than one-third of adults in the United States are obese [1]. Obese children are at risk of becoming obese adults [2] and can experience immediate health consequences such as psychosocial stress, elevated blood pressure and cholesterol, and abnormal glucose tolerance [3]. Monitoring trends in childhood obesity is important in order to assess interventions aimed at reducing the burden of obesity.

Keywords: Canadian Health Measures Survey, body mass index, international comparison, National Health and Nutrition Examination Survey

Have Changes in Obesity Prevalence in the Last 30 Years Been Similar in Canada and the United States?

During the late 1970s, there was no difference between Canada and the United States in the prevalence of childhood obesity (approximately 5% in both countries) (Figure 1). An increasing trend in childhood obesity has been seen in both countries, but the increase was greater in the United States. Beginning in the early part of the 21st century, the prevalence of childhood obesity was approximately 4 percentage points lower in Canada (12.4% in 2004; 13.0% in 2009–2013) than in the United States (16.6% in 2001–2004; 17.5% in 2009–2012), although there was no significant change between the two most recent time periods in either country.

Were Differences by Age Seen in the Prevalence of Childhood Obesity Between Canada and the United States?

Among children aged 7–12, the prevalence of obesity was more than 7 percentage points lower in Canada compared with the United States (11.8% in Canada and 19.2% in the United States) (Figure 2).

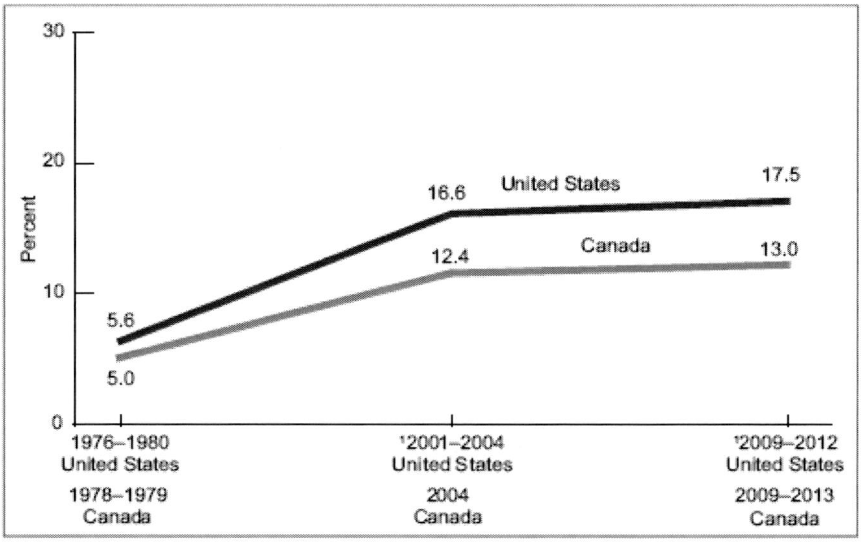

Sources: CDC/NCHS, National Health and Nutrition Examination Surveys, 1976–1980, 2001–2004, and 2009–2012; Canada Health, 1978–1979; Canadian Community Health Survey—Nutrition 2004; and Canadian Health Measures Survey, 2009–2013.

Note: Pregnant girls are excluded.

[1] Statistically significant difference compared with Canada, $p < 0.001$.

Figure 2. Childhood obesity among children and adolescents aged 3–19, by age: Canada, 2009–2013, and United States, 2009–2012.

For children aged 3–6 and adolescents aged 13–19, there were no significant differences in the prevalence of obesity in Canada and United States. For adolescents aged 13–19, the sample size may not have been large enough to detect a difference.

WERE DIFFERENCES BY SEX AND AGE SEEN IN THE PREVALENCE OF CHILDHOOD OBESITY BETWEEN CANADA AND THE UNITED STATES?

Overall, among children and adolescents aged 3–19, the prevalence of obesity among girls was significantly lower in Canada than in the United States (10.4% compared with 16.7%) but not for Canadian boys (Figure 3). Among the youngest children (3–6 years), there was no significant difference in obesity prevalence between Canada and the United States for either boys or girls.

Canadian boys (14.8%) and girls (8.7%) aged 7–12 had a lower prevalence of obesity than their U.S. counterparts (20.0% for boys, 18.5% for girls). Among adolescent boys aged 13–19, there was no significant difference in obesity prevalence, but among girls of this age group, the prevalence of obesity was lower in Canada (11.7%) than in the United States (18.3%).

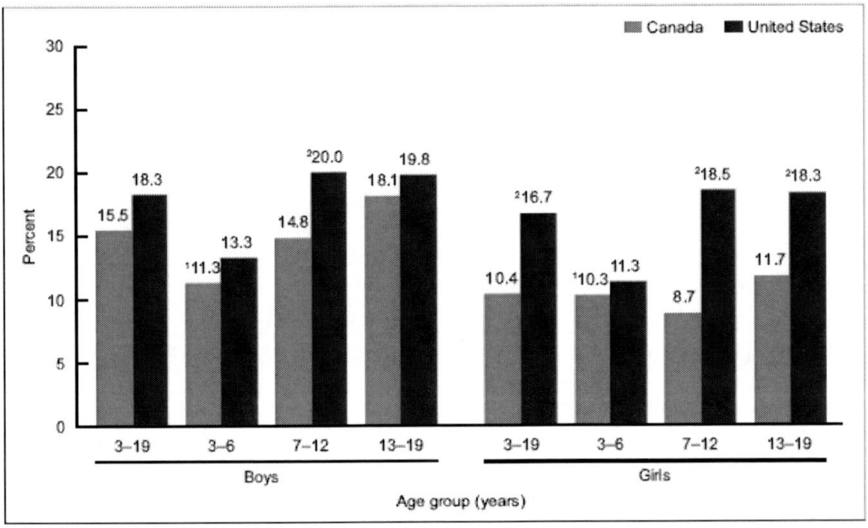

Sources: CDC/NCHS, National Health and Nutrition Examination Survey, 2009–2012, and Canadian Health Measures Survey, 2009–2013.

Note: Pregnant girls are excluded.

[1] Use with caution (coefficient of variation between 16.6% and 33.3% for the Canadian Health Measures Survey). The coefficient of variation is obtained by dividing the standard error of the estimate by the estimate itself, and it is expressed as a percentage of the estimate.

[2] Statistically significant difference compared with Canada, $p < 0.001$.

Figure 3. Childhood obesity among children and adolescents aged 3–19, by sex and age: Canada, 2009–2013, and United States, 2009–2012.

Were Differences Seen in the Prevalence of Childhood Obesity Among the Non-Hispanic White Population Between Canada and the United States?

Among non-Hispanic white boys aged 3–19, there was no significant difference between Canada and the United States in the prevalence of obesity (Figure 4). Similar to the overall population, the prevalence of childhood obesity among non-Hispanic white girls was lower in Canada than in the United States (10.2% compared with 14.2%). But when stratified by age group, only Canadian girls aged 7–12 had a significantly lower prevalence of obesity than their U.S. counterparts (8.8% compared with 15.2%).

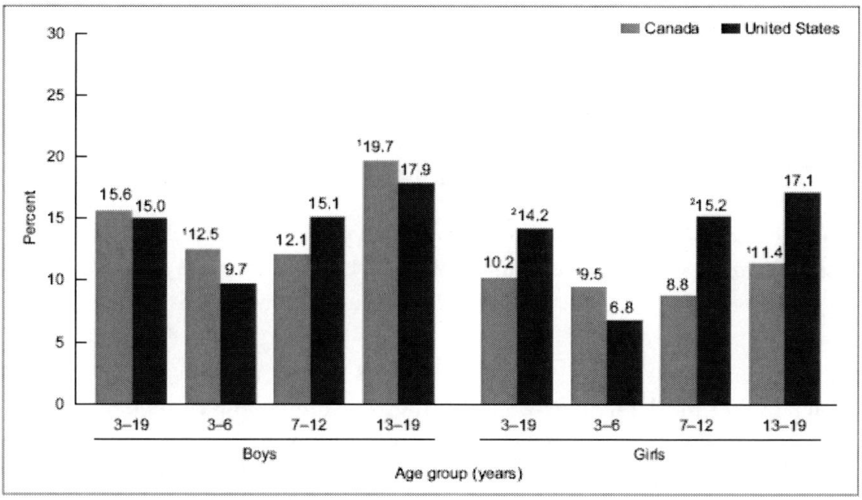

Sources: CDC/NCHS, National Health and Nutrition Examination Survey, 2009–2012, and Canadian Health Measures Survey, 2009–2013.

Note: Pregnant girls are excluded.

[1] Use with caution (coefficient of variation between 16.6% and 33.3% for the Canadian Health Measures Survey). The coefficient of variation obtained by dividing the standard error of the estimate by the estimate itself, and it is expressed as a percentage of the estimate.

[2]Statistically significant difference compared with Canada, $p < 0.001$.

Figure 4. Childhood obesity among non-Hispanic white children and adolescents aged 3–19, by sex and age: Canada, 2009–2013, and United States, 2009–2012.

There was no difference in the prevalence of obesity between girls aged 3–6 in Canada and the United States and no significant difference for non-Hispanic white girls aged 13–19, which may be because the sample size was not large enough to detect a difference.

SUMMARY

The prevalence of childhood obesity was lower in Canada than in the United States. This difference was particularly pronounced in girls compared with boys. In analysis restricted to the non-Hispanic white population, the prevalence of obesity among boys was virtually identical in Canada and the United States (15.6% compared with 15.0%). Among non-Hispanic white girls, however, just more than 10% of girls in Canada were obese compared with a little more than 14% in the United States.

Previous comparisons of childhood obesity in Canada, Mexico, and the United States through 2004 found similar changes in childhood obesity in each of the three countries [4]. Although age, income, and education differed somewhat within each country, the prevalence had increased in all three countries.

Both Canada and the United States have seen increases in childhood obesity from 1980 to the beginning of the 21st century, and then no recent changes in prevalence. This plateau (or in some cases, a decrease) in childhood obesity prevalence has been reported in at least eight other countries [5]. Similar to childhood obesity, the prevalence of obesity among adults increased in Canada and the United States from the late 1980s and early 1990s to the first decade of the 21st century [1].

Future data from the National Health and Nutrition Examination Survey (NHANES) and the Canadian Health Measures Survey (CHMS) will provide information on the direction of trends in obesity among youth in Canada and the United States.

DEFINITIONS

Body mass index (BMI): Weight in kilograms divided by height in meters squared, rounded to the nearest 10th.

Obesity: BMI at or above the sex-specific 95th percentile of BMI for age, based on the 2000 CDC (Centers for Disease Control and Prevention) Growth Charts.

Non-Hispanic white: In Canada, all respondents were asked the question: "People living in Canada come from many different cultural and racial backgrounds. Are you: white, Chinese, South Asian, Black, Filipino, Latin American, South East Asian, Arab, West Asian, Japanese, Korean, or Other?" Respondents could select more than one answer. Respondents who answered only white were used for the analysis on non-Hispanic white children and adolescents.

In the United States, non-Hispanic white was defined based on combining participant responses to questions on race and Hispanic origin. Participants were asked if they identified themselves as Hispanic and which of the following races they considered themselves (choosing one or more): American Indian or Alaska Native, Asian, black or African American, Native Hawaiian or Pacific Islander, white, or other. Respondents who answered only white and did not identify as Hispanic were considered non-Hispanic white.

DATA SOURCES AND METHODS

Canadian estimates are based on data from three cross-sectional surveys: the 1978–1979 Canada Health Survey (CHS), the 2004 Canadian Community Health Survey–Nutrition (CCHS–Nutrition), and cycles 2 and 3 (2009–2013) of CHMS [6]. These surveys were designed to provide nationally representative estimates of the Canadian noninstitutionalized population [7, 8]. In addition to an interview, these surveys included direct measurement of height and weight either at the home (CCHS and CHS) or in a mobile examination center (CHMS). Measured height and weight data for individuals aged 3–19 were available on 1,974 youths in CHS, 8,994 in CCHS–Nutrition, and 5,334 in CHMS.

United States estimates are based on data from three cycles of NHANES: NHANES II (1976– 1980), NHANES 2001–2004, and NHANES 2009–2012. NHANES, conducted by the Centers for Disease Control and Prevention's (CDC) National Center for Health Statistics (NCHS), is designed to monitor the health and nutritional status of the United States civilian noninstitutionalized population [9], using highly stratified multistage probability designs. The survey consists of interviews conducted in participants' homes and standardized physical examinations conducted in mobile examination centers, including measured height and weight. Standardized measurements of height and weight for youth aged 3–19 were collected from 6,687 participants in NHANES II, 7,742 in NHANES 2001–2004, and 6,233 in NHANES 2009–2012.

For all surveys, sample weights—which account for the differential probabilities of selection, nonresponse, and noncoverage—are incorporated into the estimation process. For CHS, standard errors were estimated under the assumption of simple random sampling. For CCHS–Nutrition and CHMS, standard errors of the prevalence of obesity were estimated using the bootstrap method [10]. For NHANES, standard errors were estimated by Taylor series linearization [10]. Both the bootstrap and Taylor series linearization methods account for the design features of the survey. To compare the prevalence of obesity between Canada and the United States, statistical hypotheses were tested using Student's t statistic and an α level of 0.05. All differences reported are statistically significant unless otherwise indicated. Linear trends in obesity prevalence over time were tested using orthogonal contrast matrices. Statistical analyses were conducted using SAS release 9.3 (SAS Institute, Inc., Cary, N.C.) and SUDAAN software version 11.0 (RTI International, Research Triangle Park, N.C.).

About the Authors

Margaret D. Carroll is with CDC's National Center for Health Statistics; Tanya Navaneelan and Shirley Bryan are with Statistics Canada; and Cynthia L. Ogden is with the National Center for Health Statistics.

References

[1] Shields M, Carroll MD, Ogden CL. Adult obesity prevalence in Canada and the United States. NCHS data brief, no 56. Hyattsville, MD: National Center for Health Statistics. 2011.

[2] Singh AS, Mulder C, Twisk JW, van Mechelen W, Chinapaw MJ. Tracking of childhood overweight into adulthood: A systematic review of the literature. *Obes. Rev.* 9(5):474–88. 2008.

[3] Barlow SE, Expert Committee. Expert Committee recommendations regarding the prevention, assessment, and treatment of child and adolescent overweight and obesity: Summary report. *Pediatrics* 120(Suppl. 4)S164–92. 2007.

[4] Ogden CL, Connor Gorber S, Rivera Dommarco JA, Carroll M, Shields M, Flegal K. Chapter 5: The epidemiology of childhood obesity in Canada, Mexico and the United States. In: Moreno LA, Pigeot I, Ahrens W (editors). Epidemiology of obesity in children and adolescents: Prevalence and etiology. New York, NY: Springer Science+Business Media, LLC. 2011.

[5] Olds T, Maher C, Zumin S, Péneau S, Lioret S, Castetbon K, et al. Evidence that the prevalence of childhood overweight is plateauing: Data from nine countries. *Int. J. Pediatr. Obes.* 6(5–6): 342–60. 2011.

[6] Statistics Canada. List of other Canadian Health Measures Survey (CHMS) documents available. Available from: http://www23.statcan.gc.ca/imdb-bmdi/document/5071_D4_T9_V2- eng.htm.

[7] Statistics Canada. Canadian Community Health Survey–Nutrition. Available from: http://www23.statcan.gc.ca/imdb/p2SV.pl?Function=getSurvey&SDDS=5049.

[8] Giroux S. Canadian Health Measures Survey: Sampling strategy overview. Health Rep 18(Suppl):31–6. 2007.

[9] NCHS. National Health and Nutrition Examination Survey: Questionnaires, datasets, and related documentation. Available from: http://www.cdc.gov/nchs/nhanes/nhanes_questionnaires. htm.

[10] Wolter KM. Introduction to variance estimation. 2nd ed. New York, NY: Springer Science+Business Media, LLC. 2007.

In: Significant Health Statistics
Editor: Christopher Barrett
ISBN: 978-1-63484-563-2

Chapter 9

SEXUAL ACTIVITY, CONTRACEPTIVE USE, AND CHILDBEARING OF TEENAGERS AGED 15–19 IN THE UNITED STATES*

Gladys M. Martinez, PhD, and Joyce C. Abma, PhD

KEY FINDINGS

Data from the 2011–2013 National Survey of Family Growth

- In 2011–2013, 44% of female teenagers and 47% of male teenagers aged 15–19 had experienced sexual intercourse; the percentage has declined significantly, by 14% for female and 22% for male teenagers, over the past 25 years.
- In the early teen years males were more likely than females to have had sexual intercourse. But the percentage of older teenagers who had sexual intercourse was similar for female and male teenagers.
- In 2011–2013, 79% of female teenagers and 84% of male teenagers used a contraceptive method at first sexual intercourse.
- The condom remained the most common contraceptive method used among teenagers.

---

* This is an edited, reformatted and augmented version of NCHS Data Brief No. 209, issued by the National Center for Health Statistics, July 2015.

- Young women who did not use a method of contraception at first sexual intercourse were twice as likely to become teen mothers as those who used a method.

Monitoring sexual activity and contraceptive use among U.S. adolescents is important for understanding differences in their risk of pregnancy. In 2013, the U.S. birth rate for teenagers aged 15–19 dropped 57% from its peak in 1991 [1], paralleling a decline in the teen *pregnancy* rate [1–2]. But these rates are still higher than those in other developed countries [3–4]. Using data from the 1988 to 2011–2013 National Survey of Family Growth (NSFG), this report provides trends and recent national estimates of sexual activity, contraceptive use, and childbearing among teenagers aged 15–19.

Keywords: adolescents, sexual intercourse, contraceptive use at first sex, National Survey of Family Growth

WHAT PERCENTAGE OF TEENAGERS AGED 15–19 HAD SEXUAL INTERCOURSE AT LEAST ONCE?

- In 2011–2013, 44% of never-married female teenagers (4.3 million) and 47% of never-married male teenagers (4.8 million) had sexual intercourse at least once (Figure 1).
- The percentage of female teenagers who had sex at least once declined 14%, from 51% in 1988 to 43% in 2006–2010. The percentage in 2006–2010 was similar to that in 2011–2013 (44%).
- Among male teenagers, there was a significant linear decline in the percentage who had sexual intercourse at least once between 1988 (60%) and 2002 (46%). However, there was no significant change in the percentage of male teenagers who had sexual intercourse at least once between 2002 and 2011–2013 (46% to 47%).

WHAT IS THE PROBABILITY OF HAVING HAD SEXUAL INTERCOURSE BY AGES 15–19?

- In the early teen years (ages 15 and 16) males were more likely than females to have had sexual intercourse (Figure 2). By age 17, the probabilities of having had sexual intercourse were similar for males and females.

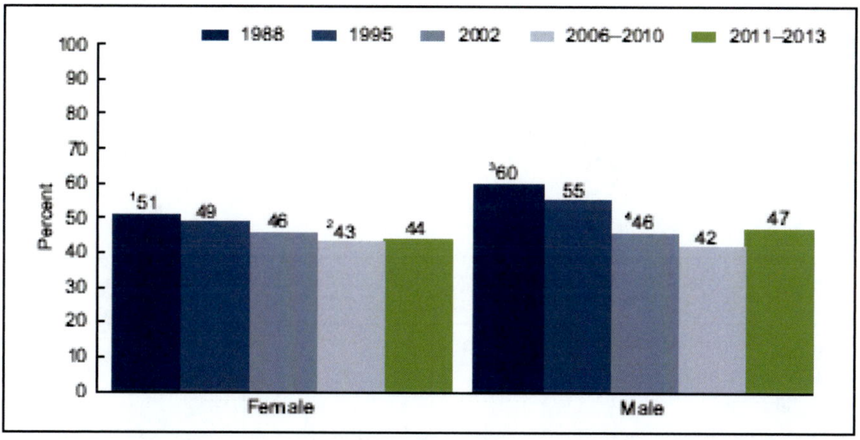

Sources: CDC/NCHS, National Survey of Family Growth, 1988, 1995, 2002, 2006–2010, and 2011–2013. Male data for 1988 and 1995 is from the National Survey of Adolescent Males.

[1] The decline in the percentage of female teenagers who had sex at least once from 1988 to 2006–2010 was statistically significant ($p < 0.05$).

[2] The difference in the percentages between 2006–2010 and 2011–2013 was not significant.

[3] The decline in the percentage of male teenagers who had sexual intercourse at least once from 1988 to 2002 was statistically significant ($p < 0.05$).

[4] There was no significant change in the percentage between 2002 and 2011–2013.

Figure 1. Never-married females and males aged 15–19 who have ever had sexual intercourse: United States, 1988–2013.

- For males, by age 15, 18% had ever had sexual intercourse. By age 17, this percentage increased to 44%, and by age 19, 69% of males had ever had sexual intercourse.
- For females, by age 15, 13% had ever had sexual intercourse. By age 17, this percentage increased to 43%, and by age 19, 68% of females had ever had sexual intercourse.

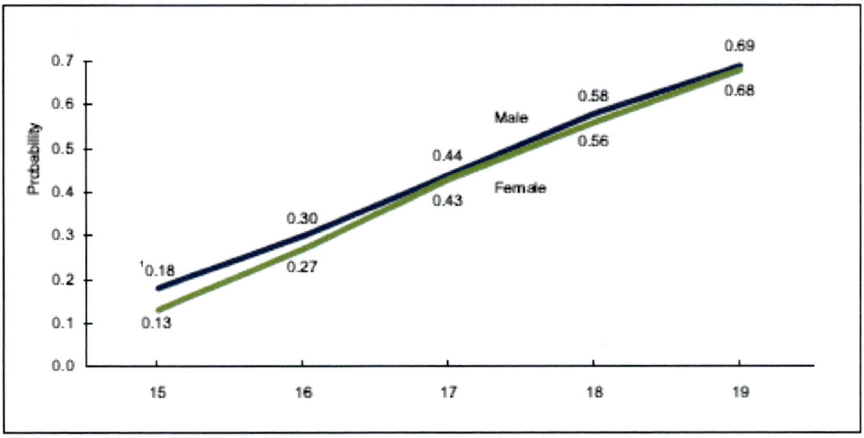

Source: CDC/NCHS, National Survey of Family Growth, 2011–2013.

Note: The estimates are based on females and males aged 15–24 at the time of the interview.

[1] Male teenagers have a higher probability of having had sex at each age in teen years compared to female teenagers, except for ages 17 and 19 ($p < 0.05$).

Figure 2. Probability of having had sex by ages 15, 16, 17, 18, and 19 for males and females: United States, 2011–2013.

Did the Percentage of Teenagers Who Used Contraceptives at First Sexual Intercourse Differ by Age at First Sexual Intercourse?

- In 2011–2013, 79% of female teenagers and 84% of male teenagers used a method of contraception the first time they had sexual intercourse (Figure 3). The percentages have not changed over time (data not shown).
- A higher percentage of female teenagers who had first sexual intercourse at ages 18 or 19 used a method of contraception (93%) compared with those who were 17 and under at first sexual intercourse (77%).
- Almost all male teenagers who had first sexual intercourse at ages 18 or 19 used a method of contraception (99%) compared with those who were 17 and under at first sexual intercourse (82%).

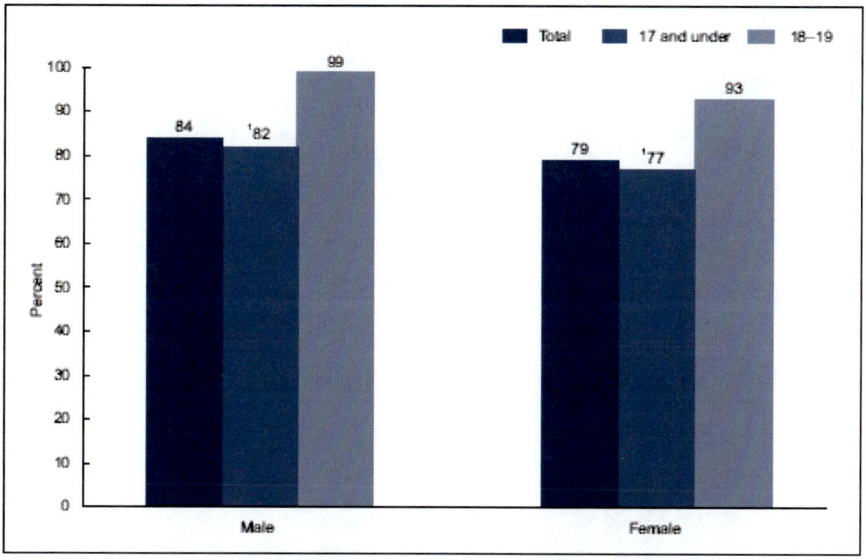

Source: CDC/NCHS, National Survey of Family Growth, 2011–2013.

[1] Percentage of male and female teenagers aged 17 and under who used contraception at first sex was significantly lower than that of teenagers aged 18–19 ($p < 0.05$).

Figure 3. Use of contraception at first sex among males and females aged 15–19, by age at first sex: United States, 2011–2013.

How Has Contraceptive Method Use Changed Over the Past Decade Among Female Teenagers Who Had Sexual Intercourse at Least Once?

- In 2011–2013, 97% of female teenagers who had sexual intercourse at least once had used the condom at least once (Figure 4).
- In 2011–2013, 60% of female teenagers had ever used withdrawal and 54% had ever used the pill. The differences in pill and withdrawal use between 2002 and 2011–2013 were not statistically significant.
- Use of emergency contraception by female teenagers who had sexual intercourse at least once has increased over the past decade from 8% in 2002 to 22% in 2011–2013.
- Compared with 2006–2010, in 2011–2013, a smaller percentage of female teenagers ever used the patch (from 10% to 2%) and ever used Depo-Provera (from 20% to 15%). As of 2011–2013, approximately

3% of female teenagers who had sexual intercourse at least once had ever used an intrauterine device (IUD), and 2% had used a hormonal implant, similar to the percentages in 2006–2010.

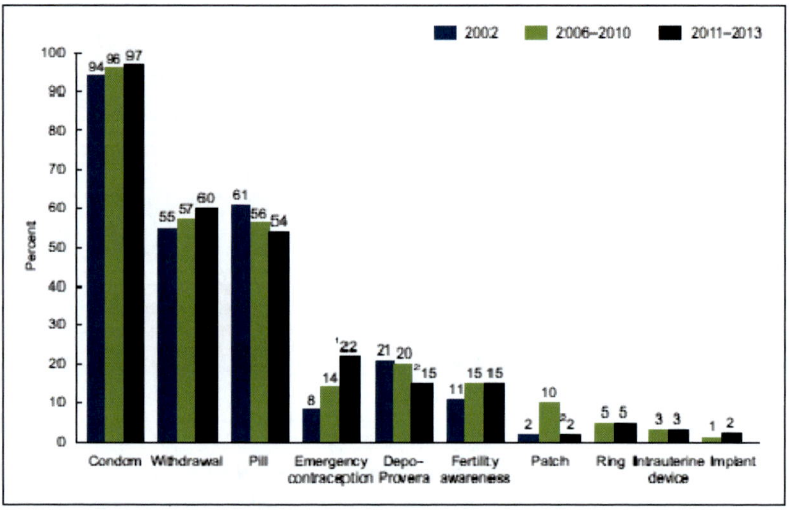

Source: CDC/NCHS, National Survey of Family Growth, 2002, 2006–2010, and 2011–2013.

[1] The percentage of female teenagers who ever used emergency contraception increased in 2006–2010 and in 2011–2013 ($p < 0.05$).2Difference in percentage of female teenagers who ever used Depo-Provera or the patch was significantly lower in 2011–2013 than in 2006–2010 ($p < 0.05$).NOTES: Neither the contraceptive ring nor the implant were available in 2002. The number of teenagers who had ever used the IUD in 2002 was too small to be statistically reliable.

Figure 4. Methods of contraception ever used among females aged 15–19 who had ever had sexual intercourse: United States, 2002, 2006–2010, and 2011–2013.

Were Female Teenagers Who Didn't Use a Method of Contraception at First Sexual Intercourse More Likely to Have Had a Birth as a Teenager Than Those Who Used a Method?

- By age 17, young women were more than five times as likely to have had a teen birth if they did not use a method of contraception at their first sexual intercourse (11%) than those who used a method (2%) (Figure 5).

- By age 18, young women were more than three times as likely to have had a teen birth if they did not use a method of contraception at their first sexual intercourse (17%) than those who used a method (5%).
- By age 19, young women were more than twice as likely to have had a teen birth if they did not use a method of contraception at their first sexual intercourse (26%) than those who used a method (10%).

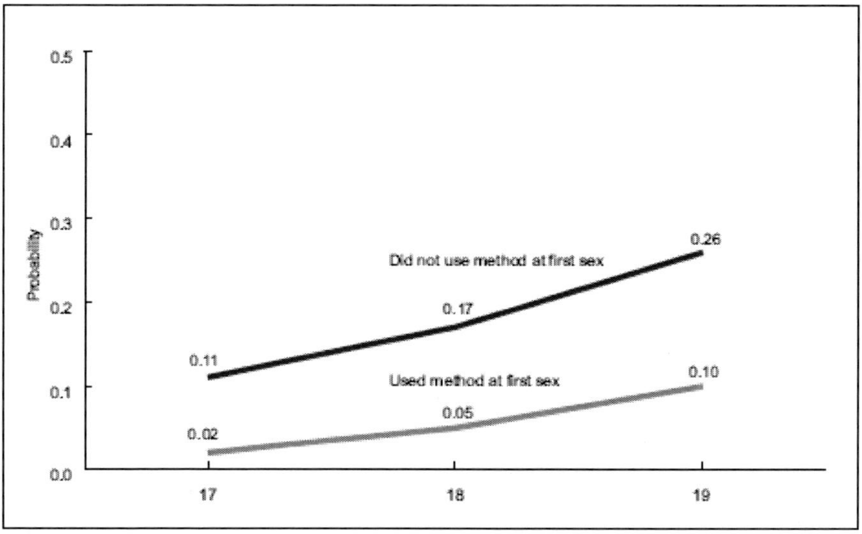

Source: CDC/NCHS, National Survey of Family Growth, 2011-2013.
Note: The estimates are based on females aged 15–24 at the time of the interview.

Figure 5. Probability of a first birth by ages 17, 18, and 19 for females, by whether they used a method of contraception at first sex: United States, 2011–2013.

SUMMARY

This report updates selected indicators of sexual activity, contraceptive use, and childbearing among the teenage population in the United States using the most recent NSFG data available. In addition to costing the public about $9.4 billion a year [5], teen childbearing has negative consequences for the physical, psychological, and economic wellbeing of the young mothers and their children [6–8]. The percentage of male and female teenagers who had sexual intercourse at least once has declined in the 25-year period of 1988 to 2013. This decline was greater for male teenagers than female teenagers. According to the most recent data from 2011–2013, by age 19, roughly two of three never-married teenagers have had sexual intercourse. The majority of male and female teenagers used a method of contraception at first sexual intercourse. The methods teenagers most often used were the condom, withdrawal, and the oral contraceptive pill. Female teenagers who used a method of contraception at first sexual intercourse were less likely to have had a birth in their teen years than those who did not use a method of contraception at first intercourse. Understanding these patterns and trends in sexual activity, contraceptive use, and their impact on teen pregnancy can help provide context regarding the recent decline in the U.S. teen birth rate.

DEFINITIONS

Age at first sexual intercourse: The recode variable VRY1STAG indicates the respondent's age at first sexual intercourse, even if it was before a female respondent's menarche (age at first menstrual period).

Age at first birth: The recode variable AGEBABY1 indicates the female respondent's age at her first live birth, if any.

Contraceptive methods ever used: These data are based on a series of yes or no questions asking the female respondent if she has ever used each of 19 different contraceptive methods. The following are the contraceptive methods included in this series: the pill; condom; partner's vasectomy; Depo-Provera injectable; withdrawal; fertility awareness-based methods (e.g., rhythm method or natural family planning); contraceptive patch; contraceptive ring; emergency contraception; hormonal implant; IUD; cervical cap; diaphragm; female condom or vaginal pouch; foam; jelly or cream; suppository or insert; Today sponge; and other method.

Probability of first birth by selected ages: The probability that an individual has had a first birth by various ages was calculated using a life table methodology. This methodology uses age-specific rates to calculate how many individuals of a cohort will experience an event (i.e., first birth) during an interval. The probabilities produced by life table methodology do not represent the actual percentages of individuals who have had a baby by each age shown; instead, they represent how likely it is that an individual will have a baby by a specified age, given the age-specific first birth rates observed for this NSFG-based cohort. For example, a probability of first birth of 0.26 by age 19 means that by age 19 there is a 26% probability that young females will have had a baby.

Probability of first sexual intercourse by selected ages: The probability that an individual has experienced his or her first sexual intercourse by various ages was calculated using a life table methodology. This methodology uses age-specific rates to calculate how many individuals of a cohort will experience an event (i.e., first sexual intercourse) during an interval. The probabilities produced by life table methodology do not represent the actual percentages of individuals who have had sex by each age shown; instead, they represent how likely it is that an individual will have sex by a specified age, given the age-specific first sex rates observed for this NSFG-based cohort. For example, a probability of first sex of 0.78 by age 20 for males means that by age 20 there is a 78% probability that young males will have experienced sex for the first time.

Sexual experience: The recode variable HADSEX indicates whether the respondent ever had vaginal sexual intercourse, referred to in this report simply as sexual intercourse.

Used a contraceptive method at first sexual intercourse: The recode variable SEX1MTHD1 indicates whether any contraceptive method was used at first sexual intercourse, and if so, what method(s).

DATA SOURCES AND METHODS

This report is based on data from 1,037 females and 1,088 male teenagers aged 15–19. For Figures 2 and 5, analysis included an additional 960 females and 810 males aged 20–24 interviewed in the 2011–2013 NSFG. These additional cases were included to increase sample size because some teenagers aged 15–19 who have not experienced these events may do so before age 20, and adults aged 20–24 have completed their teen years and can provide information on whether they experienced these events in their teen years. Trends are presented using data from four other data collection periods of NSFG (1988, 1995, 2002, and 2006–2010).

Among other information, NSFG provides detailed information about sexual intercourse, contraceptive use, and the timing of childbearing among U.S. women aged 15–44. The fieldwork plan, interview content, and other procedures of the survey are similar to what was done in previous surveys [9]. NSFG is jointly planned and funded by the Centers for Disease

Control and Prevention's (CDC) National Center for Health Statistics and several other programs of the U.S. Department of Health and Human Services. All estimates in this report were weighted to reflect the female and male teenage household population of the United States across the midpoint of 2011–2013 interviewing (July 2012). The response rate for both female and male teenagers in 2011–2013 was 75%.

Statistics for this report were produced using the SURVEY procedures in SAS software version 9.3. The probabilities of first sexual intercourse (Figure 2) and first birth (Figure 5) were produced using the PROC LIFETEST procedure in SAS. Percentages were compared using two-tailed *t* tests at the 5% level. No adjustments were made for multiple comparisons. The data presented in this report are bivariate associations that may be explained by other factors not controlled for in the figures or included in the report.

About the Authors

Gladys M. Martinez and Joyce C. Abma are with CDC's National Center for Health Statistics, Division of Vital Statistics, Reproductive Statistics Branch.

References

[1] Martin JA, Hamilton BE, Osterman MJK, et al. Births: Final data for 2013. National vital statistics reports; vol 64 no 1. Hyattsville, MD: National Center for Health Statistics. 2015.

[2] Kost K, Henshaw S. U.S. teenage pregnancies, births and abortions, 2010: National and state trends by age, race and ethnicity. 2014. Available from: http://www.guttmacher.org/pubs/USTPtrends10.pdf.

[3] HHS. Healthy People. 2020 topics and objectives: Family planning. Washington, DC. Available from: http://www.healthypeople.gov/2020/topicsobjectives/topic/family-planning.

[4] CDC. CDC winnable battles 2010–2015: Progress report 2014. Available from: http://www.cdc.gov/winnablebattles/targets/pdf/winnablebattles2010-2015_progressreport2014_.pdf.

[5] The National Campaign to Prevent Teen and Unplanned Pregnancy. Teen childbearing cost taxpayers $9.4 billion in 2010. 2013. Available from: https://thenationalcampaign.org/press-release/teen-childbearing-cost-taxpayers94-billion-2010.

[6] Jutte DP, Roos NP, Brownell MD, Briggs G, MacWilliam L, Roos LL. The ripples of adolescent motherhood: Social, educational, and medical outcomes for children of teen and prior teen mothers. *Acad. Pediatr.* 10(5):293–301. 2010.

[7] Lee D. The early socioeconomic effects of teenage childbearing: A propensity score matching approach. *Demographic Research* 23(25):697–736. 2010.

[8] Hoffman S, Maynard R. Kids having kids: Economic costs and social consequences of teen pregnancy. 2nd edition. Washington, DC: The Urban Institute Press. 2008.

[9] Lepkowski JM, Mosher WD, Davis KE, et al. The 2006–2010 National Survey of Family Growth: Sample design and analysis of a continuous survey. National Center for Health Statistics. Vital Health Stat 2(150). 2010. Available from: http://www.cdc.gov/nchs/data/series/sr_02/sr02_150.pdf.

In: Significant Health Statistics
Editor: Christopher Barrett
ISBN: 978-1-63484-563-2

Chapter 10

SERIOUS PSYCHOLOGICAL DISTRESS AMONG ADULTS: UNITED STATES, 2009–2013*

Judith Weissman, PhD, Laura A. Pratt, PhD, Eric A. Miller, PhD, and Jennifer D. Parker, PhD

KEY FINDINGS

Data from the National Health Interview Survey, 2009–2013

- In every age group, women were more likely to have serious psychological distress than men.
- Among all adults, as income increased, the percentage with serious psychological distress decreased.
- Adults aged 18–64 with serious psychological distress were more likely to be uninsured (30.4%) than adults without serious psychological distress (20.5%).
- More than one-quarter of adults aged 65 and over with serious psychological distress (27.3%) had limitations in activities of daily living.

* This is an edited, reformatted and augmented version of NCHS Data Brief No. 203, issued by the National Center for Health Statistics, May 2015.

- Adults with serious psychological distress were more likely to have chronic obstructive pulmonary disease, heart disease, and diabetes than adults without serious psychological distress.

Serious psychological distress includes mental health problems severe enough to cause moderate-to-serious impairment in social, occupational, or school functioning and to require treatment [1]. Data from the 2009–2013 National Health Interview Survey (NHIS) are used to estimate the prevalence of serious psychological distress—measured by a score of 13 or greater on the Kessler 6 (K6) nonspecific distress scale—among adults overall and by demographic characteristics. The K6 obtains information on the frequency of six psychological distress symptoms [2]. This report also compares health insurance and health characteristics between those with and those without serious psychological distress.

Keywords: mental health, health insurance coverage, poverty, National Health Interview Survey

In Every Age Group, Women Were More Likely to Have Serious Psychological Distress Than Men

Among adults aged 18 and over, 3.4% had serious psychological distress, including 3.9% of women and 2.8% of men (Figure 1).

Adults aged 45–64 were more likely to have serious psychological distress (4.3%) than adults aged 18–44 (3.1%) or adults aged 65 and over (2.4%).

As Income Increased, the Age-Adjusted Percentage with Serious Psychological Distress Decreased

A total of 8.7% of adults with income below the federal poverty level had serious psychological distress, compared with 1.2% of adults with incomes at or above 400% of the poverty level (Figure 2).

Serious psychological distress affects 3.3% of non-Hispanic white, 3.7% of non-Hispanic black, and 3.8% of Hispanic adults.

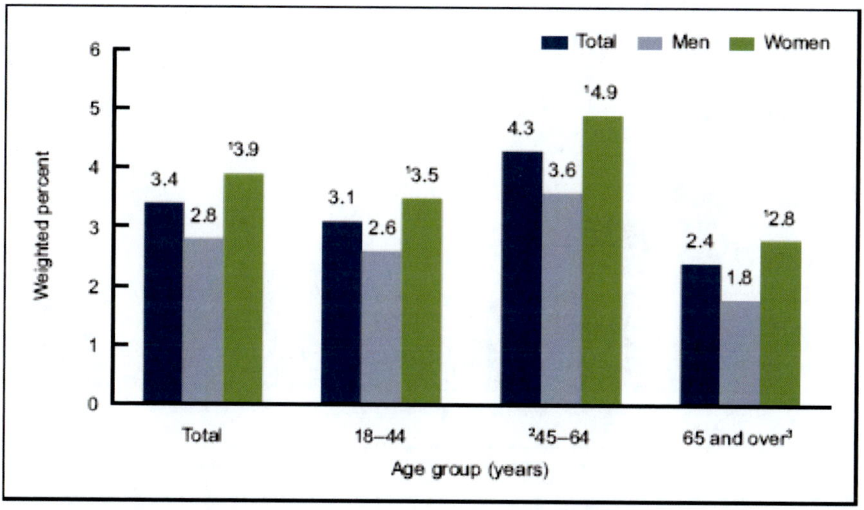

Source: CDC/NCHS, National Health Interview Survey, 2009–2013.

[1]Significantly higher percentage of women with serious psychological distress than men.

[2]Significantly higher percentage with serious psychological distress than other age groups.

[3]Significantly lower percentage with serious psychological distress than other age groups.

Figure 1. Percentage of adults aged 18 and over at interview with serious psychological distress, by sex and age: United States, 2009–2013.

The age-adjusted percentage of non-Hispanic white adults with serious psychological distress was lower compared with non-Hispanic black and Hispanic adults.

Adults Aged 18–64 with Serious Psychological Distress Were More Likely to Be Uninsured Than Adults Without Serious Psychological Distress

Among adults aged 18–64, 30.4% with serious psychological distress were uninsured compared with 20.5% without serious psychological distress (Figure 3).

In age group 18–44, 37.4% of adults with serious psychological distress were uninsured, compared with 23.5% of adults aged 45–64.

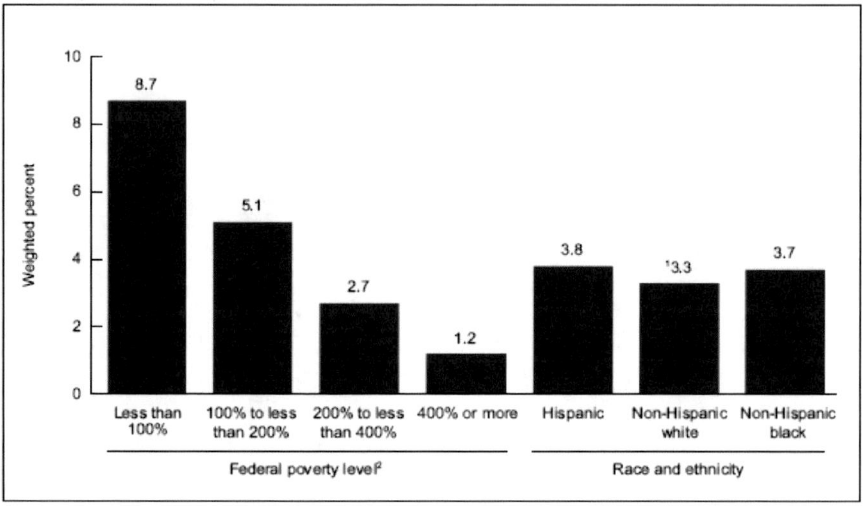

Source: CDC/NCHS, National Health Interview Survey, 2009-2013.

[1] Significantly lower than for other races and ethnicities.

[2] Significant decreasing linear trend by poverty level.

Figure 2. Age-adjusted percentage of adults with serious psychological distress, by income relative to federal poverty level and by race and ethnicity: United States, 2009–2013.

In both age groups, the percentage uninsured was higher among adults with serious psychological distress than among those without the condition.

More Than One-Quarter of Adults Aged 65 and Over With Serious Psychological Distress Had Limitations in Activities of Daily Living

Within the adult noninstitutionalized population, with or without serious psychological distress, the percentage with limitations in activities of daily living (ADL) increased with age (Figure 4).

Among adults aged 18–44, those with serious psychological distress were more than 10 times as likely to have ADL limitations as those without serious psychological distress.

Among those aged 45–64, adults with serious psychological distress were about eight times as likely to have ADL limitations as those without serious psychological distress.

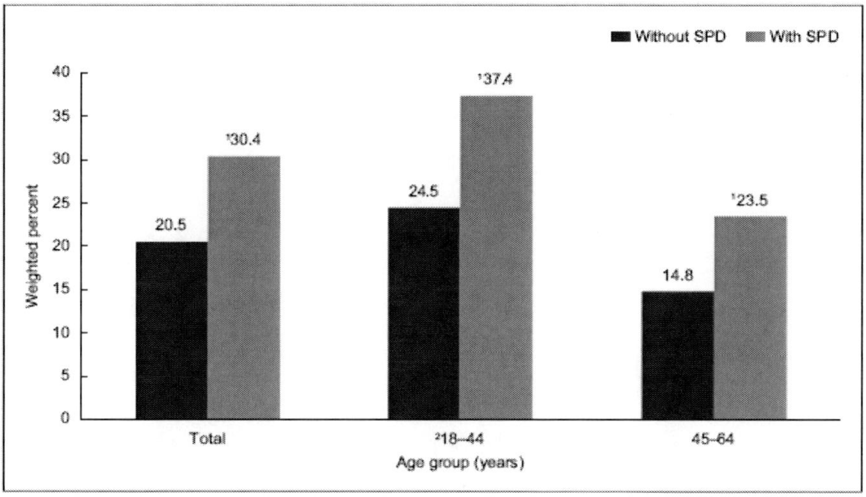

Source: CDC/NCHS, National Health Interview Survey, 2009–2013.
Note: SPD is serious psychological distress.
[1] Significant difference from adults without serious psychological distress.
[2] Significant difference in health insurance coverage compared with age group 45–64.

Figure 3. Percentage of adults aged 18–64 who were uninsured at interview, by serious psychological distress status and age: United States, 2009–2013.

Adults aged 65 and over with serious psychological distress were almost five times as likely to have ADL limitations as those without serious psychological distress in that age group.

Adults with Serious Psychological Distress Were More Likely to Have Chronic Obstructive Pulmonary Disease, Heart Disease, and Diabetes Compared with Adults Without Serious Psychological Distress

After age adjustment, men and women with serious psychological distress were approximately four times as likely to have chronic obstructive pulmonary disease (COPD) as men and women without serious psychological distress (Figure 5).

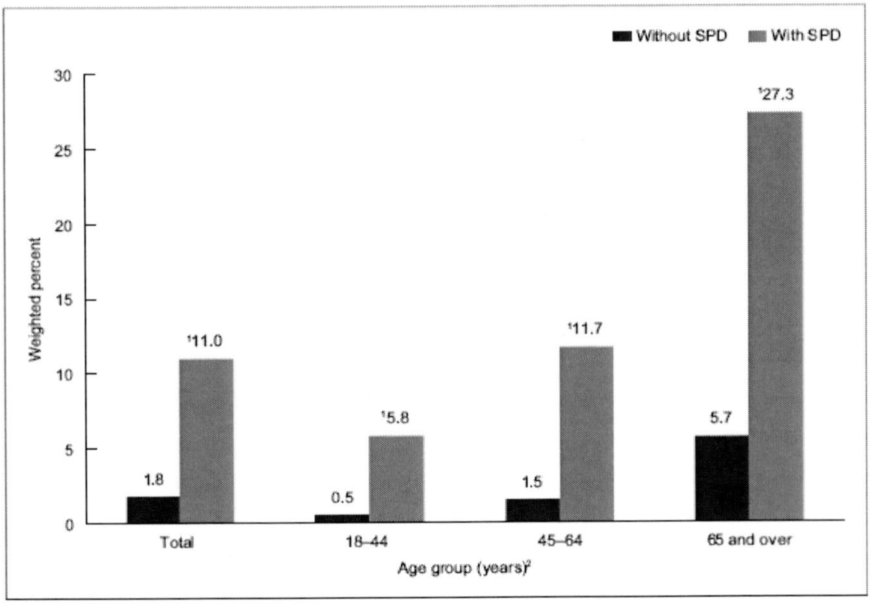

Source: CDC/NCHS, National Health Interview Survey, 2009–2013.
Note: SPD is serious psychological distress.
[1] Significant difference from adults without serious psychological distress. 2Significant increasing linear trend by age group.

Figure 4. Percentage of adults aged 18 and over with limitations in activities of daily living at interview, by serious psychological distress status and age: United States, 2009–2013.

Men and women with serious psychological distress were approximately twice as likely after age adjustment to have either heart disease or diabetes as men and women without serious psychological distress.

SUMMARY

During 2009–2013, 3.3% of the civilian noninstitutionalized population aged 18 and over had serious psychological distress. The condition was most prevalent in the 45–64 age group and least prevalent in ages 65 and over. The age-adjusted percentage of adults with serious psychological distress decreased as income increased relative to the federal poverty level.

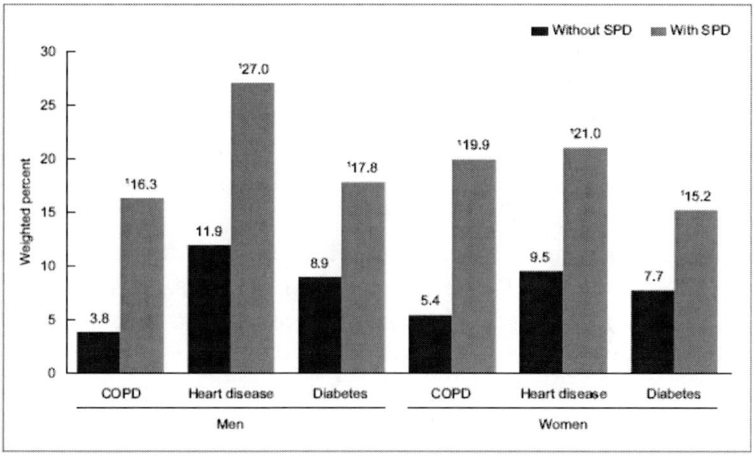

Source: CDC/NCHS, National Health Interview Survey, 2009–2013.

Notes: Disease categories are not mutually exclusive. COPD is chronic obstructive pulmonary disease. SPD is serious psychological distress.

[1] Significant difference from adults without serious psychological distress.

Figure 5. Age-adjusted percentage of adults aged 18 and over with COPD, heart disease, or diabetes at interview, by serious psychological distress status and sex: United States, 2009–2013.

Adults with serious psychological distress were more likely not to have health insurance than those without serious psychological distress, and adults aged 18–44 with serious psychological distress were more often uninsured compared with those aged 45–64. More than one-quarter of adults aged 65 and over with serious psychological distress had ADL limitations; by comparison, approximately 6% of those in the same age group without serious psychological distress had such limitations. Those aged 18 and over with serious psychological distress were more likely to have ADL limitations, and to have COPD, heart disease, or diabetes, than adults without serious psychological distress.

DEFINITIONS

Age-adjusted estimates: Prevalence estimates for race, Hispanic origin, and chronic condition categories were age-adjusted to the 2000 U.S. census population using the direct method for age groups 18–44, 45–64, and 65 and over [3].

Chronic obstructive pulmonary disease (COPD): Defined by the American Thoracic Society as a preventable and treatable disease state characterized by airflow limitation that is not fully reversible. COPD is based on separate self-reported responses to survey questions about whether the respondents had been told by a doctor or other health professional that they had chronic bronchitis in the past 12 months or ever had emphysema [4].

Diabetes: Based on self-reported responses to survey questions about whether the respondents had ever been told by a doctor or other health professional that they had diabetes or sugar diabetes. Respondents who reported having borderline diabetes were not considered to have diabetes.

Heart disease: Based on self-reported responses to survey questions about whether the respondents had ever been told by a doctor or other health professional that they had coronary heart disease, angina (angina pectoris), a heart attack (myocardial infarction), or any other kind of heart disease or heart condition.

Insurance coverage: Adults covered by private, public, or military insurance were considered to have health insurance. Persons without private, public, or military insurance, and those with only Indian Health Service coverage or only a private plan that paid for one type of service such as accidents or dental care, were considered uninsured. The years included in this analysis, 2009–2013, overlap with the Affordable Care Act's dependent coverage provision in 2010, which increased insurance coverage within age group 19–25 [5].

Limitations in activities of daily living (ADL): Defined by answering "yes" to the survey question, "Because of a physical, mental, or emotional problem, (do you/does anyone in the family) need the help of other persons with PERSONAL CARE NEEDS, such as eating, bathing, dressing, or getting around inside this home?"

Serious psychological distress: Defined as having a score greater than or equal to 13 on the Kessler 6 (K6) nonspecific distress scale [2]. The six-question K6 was developed to identify persons with a high likelihood of having a diagnosable mental illness and associated functional limitations, using as few questions as possible. The K6 asks about the frequency of each of the six symptoms of mental illness or nonspecific psychological distress:

> "During the PAST 30 DAYS, how often did you feel ...
>
> 1. So sad that nothing could cheer you up; 2. Nervous; 3. Restless or fidgety; 4. Hopeless; 5. That everything was an effort; and 6. Worthless."

Only participants who answered all six questions were included in the analysis. In a range of possible scores from 0–24, a calibration study found that a score of 13 was the best cut-off to balance false-positive and false-negative classification of psychological distress [2]. In 2013, the K6 questions were moved to a new Adult Selected Items section in NHIS, which may have changed how respondents answered the questions compared with earlier years.

Federal poverty level: Based on reported and imputed family income, family size, and number of children in the family, and for families with two or fewer adults, based on the age of adults in the family. For more details, see the U.S. Census Bureau website at: http://www.census.gov/hhes/ www/poverty/ poverty.html [6]. Note that NHIS asks respondents about their personal earnings and family income for the previous calendar year.

DATA SOURCE AND METHODS

Data from the 2009–2013 NHIS were used for this analysis. NHIS data were collected continuously throughout the year for the Centers for Disease Control and Prevention's (CDC) National Center for Health Statistics (NCHS) by interviewers from the U.S. Census Bureau. NHIS collects information about the health and health care of the civilian noninstitutionalized U.S. population. Interviews are conducted in respondents' homes, but follow-ups in order to complete interviews may be conducted over the telephone.

Point estimates were calculated using sample weights, and corresponding variances accounted for the complex sample design of NHIS. The Taylor series linearization method was chosen for variance estimation. All estimates shown in this report have a relative standard error less than or equal to 30%.

Overall associations for categorical variables were evaluated using chi square statistics. Differences between subgroups within a categorical variable were evaluated using univariate t statistics. Differences between percentages were evaluated using two-sided significance tests at the 0.05 level. Logistic regression and ANOVA Cochran Mantel Haenszel tests were performed to evaluate trends for age and poverty groups.

For 2009–2013, approximately 16% of NHIS respondents were missing data on family income and personal earnings. To analyze poverty status, NHIS' imputed personal earning and income files were used [7]. Appropriate statistical methods were applied to combine the estimates for these imputations. All analyses were conducted using SAS-callable SUDAAN software [8].

About the Authors

Judith Weissman, Laura A. Pratt, Eric A. Miller, and Jennifer D. Parker are with CDC's National Center for Health Statistics, Office of Analysis and Epidemiology.

References

[1] Pratt LA, Dey AN, Cohen AJ. Characteristics of adults with serious psychological distress as measured by the K6 scale: United States, 2001–04. Advance data from vital and health statistics; no 382. Hyattsville, MD: National Center for Health Statistics. 2007.

[2] Kessler RC, Barker PR, Colpe LJ, Epstein JF, Gfroerer JC, Hiripi E, et al. Screening for serious mental illness in the general population. *Arch. Gen. Psychiatry* 60(2):184–9. 2003.

[3] Klein RJ, Schoenborn CA. Age adjustment using the 2000 projected U.S. population. Healthy People 2010 Statistical Notes, no 20. Hyattsville, MD: National Center for Health Statistics. 2001.

[4] American Thoracic Society/European Respiratory Society Task Force. Standards for the diagnosis and management of patients with COPD. Version 1.2. New York, NY: American Thoracic Society. 2004.

[5] Kirzinger WK, Cohen RA, Gindi RM. Trends in insurance coverage and source of private coverage among young adults aged 19–25: United States, 2008–2012. NCHS data brief, no 137. Hyattsville, MD: National Center for Health Statistics. 2013. Available from: http://www. cdc.gov/nchs/data/ databriefs/db137.pdf.

[6] DeNavas-Walt C, Proctor BD, Smith JC. Income, poverty, and health insurance coverage in the United States: 2010. Current Population Reports, P60–239. Washington, DC: U.S. Census Bureau. 2011.

[7] Schenker N, Raghunathan TE, Chiu PL, et al. Multiple imputation of family income and personal earnings in the National Health Interview Survey: Methods and examples. Hyattsville, MD: National Center for Health Statistics. 2009.

[8] RTI International. SUDAAN (Release 11.0) [computer software]. 2008.

In: Significant Health Statistics
Editor: Christopher Barrett

ISBN: 978-1-63484-563-2

Chapter 11

RACIAL AND ETHNIC DISPARITIES IN MEN'S USE OF MENTAL HEALTH TREATMENTS*

Stephen J. Blumberg, PhD,
Tainya C. Clarke, PhD, MPH,
and Debra L. Blackwell, PhD

KEY FINDINGS

Data from the National Health Interview Survey, 2010–2013

- Nearly 9% of men (8.5%) had daily feelings of anxiety or depression. Less than one-half of them (41.0%) took medication for these feelings or had recently talked to a mental health professional.
- Racial and ethnic differences were observed only for men aged 18–44.
- Among men aged 18–44, non-Hispanic black and Hispanic men (6.1%) were less likely than non-Hispanic white men (8.5%) to report daily feelings of anxiety or depression.
- Among men aged 18–44 who had daily feelings of anxiety or depression, non-Hispanic black and Hispanic men (26.4%) were less likely than non-Hispanic white men (45.4%) to have used mental health treatments.

---

* This is an edited, reformatted and augmented version of NCHS Data Brief No. 206, issued by the National Center for Health Statistics, June 2015.

- The significant racial and ethnic disparity in treatment utilization was associated with lack of health insurance coverage.

Compared with white Americans, persons of other races in the United States are less likely to have access to and receive needed mental health care [1–4]. Few studies, however, have explored such disparities specifically among men. Mental health and treatment have traditionally received less attention for men than women, perhaps because men are less likely than women to report mental health problems and to receive services for these problems [4–7]. This report uses nationally representative data on frequency of mental health symptoms and related treatment utilization to compare men of color (that is, non-Hispanic black and Hispanic men) with non-Hispanic white men. It also explores whether racial and ethnic disparities differ by age, health insurance coverage status, and income.

Keywords: men's health, behavioral health, anxiety, depression

Nearly 9% of U.S. Men Reported Daily Feelings of Anxiety or Depression, But the Rate Differed by Race and Ethnicity

Among all men aged 18 and over, 7.7% had daily feelings of anxiety, 3.5% had daily feelings of depression, and 8.5% felt either anxious or depressed every day (Figure 1). However, non-Hispanic black and Hispanic men (7.3%) were significantly less likely than non-Hispanic white men (9.0%) to feel anxious or depressed every day.

Racial and Ethnic Differences in Daily Feelings of Anxiety or Depression Were Observed Only for Men Aged 18–44

Men aged 18–44 (7.6%) were significantly less likely than men aged 45 and over (9.4%) to have daily feelings of anxiety or depression (Figure 2). This difference was due largely to racial and ethnic differences in the younger age group.

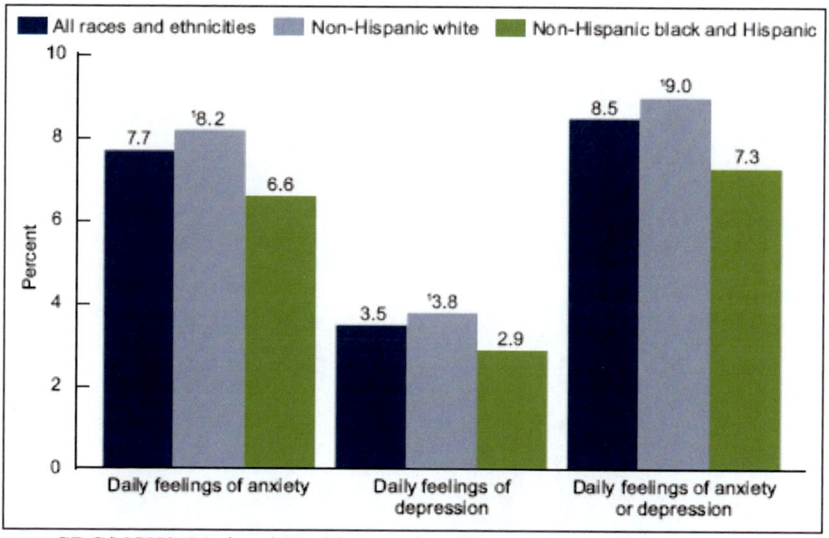

Source: CDC/NCHS, National Health Interview Survey, 2010–2013.
[1]Significantly different from non-Hispanic black and Hispanic men.

Figure 1. Men aged 18 and over with daily feelings of anxiety or depression, by race and ethnicity: United States, 2010–2013.

Among those aged 18–44, non-Hispanic black and Hispanic men (6.1%) were nearly 30% less likely than non-Hispanic white men (8.5%) to have daily feelings of anxiety or depression. Among men aged 45 and over, there were no racial or ethnic differences in the prevalence of men with daily feelings of anxiety or depression.

About 4 in 10 Men with Daily Feelings of Anxiety or Depression Took Medication for These Feelings or Talked to a Mental Health Professional, but the Rate Differed by Race and Ethnicity

One in three men (33.0%) with daily feelings of anxiety or depression took medication for those feelings, and just over one-quarter (25.7%) talked to a mental health professional within the previous 12 months (Figure 3). Among men with daily feelings of anxiety or depression, non-Hispanic white men

(43.0%) were more likely than non-Hispanic black and Hispanic men (36.0%) to have used either of these mental health treatments.

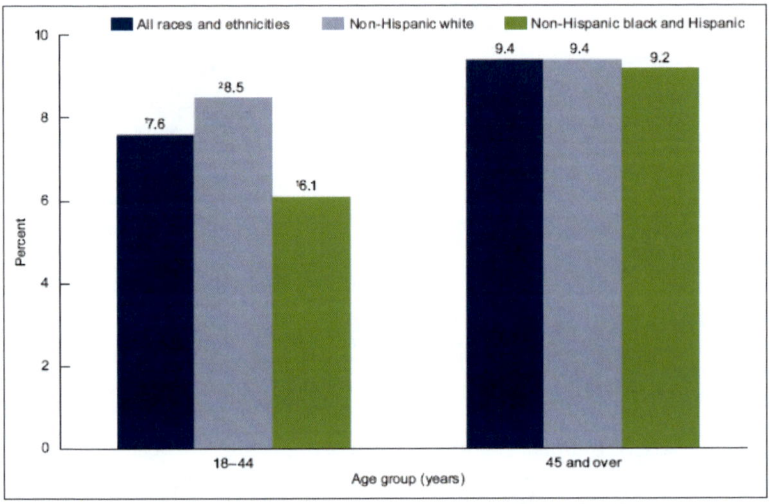

Source: CDC/NCHS, National Health Interview Survey, 2010–2013.

[1] Significantly different from men aged 45 and over in the same race and ethnicity group. 2Significantly different from non-Hispanic black and Hispanic men in the same age group.

Figure 2. Men aged 18 and over with daily feelings of anxiety or depression, by age and race and ethnicity: United States, 2010–2013.

Racial and Ethnic Differences in the Use of Mental Health Treatments by Men with Daily Feelings of Anxiety or Depression Were Observed Only for Men Aged 18–44

Among men who felt anxious or depressed on a daily basis, younger men aged 18–44 (39.2%) were as likely as older men aged 45 and over (42.3%) to have taken medication for these feelings or to have seen a mental health professional in the previous 12 months (Figure 4). However, racial and ethnic differences in the use of mental health treatments were observed among men aged 18–44 with daily feelings of anxiety or depression. In this age group, non-Hispanic black and Hispanic men (26.4%) were about 40% less likely than non-Hispanic white men (45.4%) to have used mental health treatments.

Race and ethnicity were not associated with use of mental health treatments among men aged 45 and over with daily feelings of anxiety and depression.

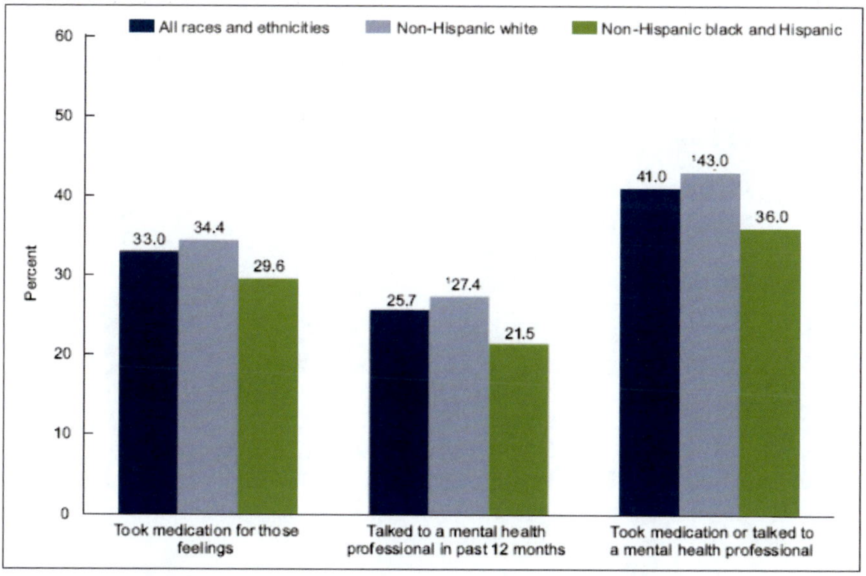

Source: CDC/NCHS, National Health Interview Survey, 2010–2013.
[1]Significantly different from non-Hispanic black and Hispanic men.

Figure 3. Men who used selected types of mental health treatments, among men aged 18 and over who felt anxious or depressed every day, by race and ethnicity: United States, 2010–2013.

Among Men Aged 18–44, Racial and Ethnic Differences in the Use of Mental Health Treatments Were Significantly Greater for Men Without Health Insurance Coverage Than for Men with Health Insurance

Among uninsured men aged 18–44 with daily feelings of anxiety or depression, non-Hispanic white men (39.3%) were three times as likely as non-Hispanic black and Hispanic men (12.7%) to have used mental health treatments (Figure 5). This disparity was significantly smaller for men aged 18–44 who had health insurance coverage.

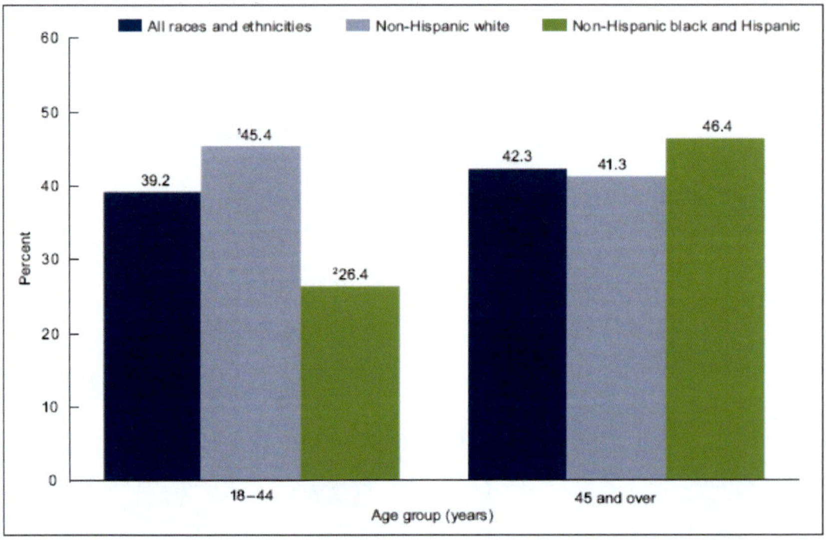

Source: CDC/NCHS, National Health Interview Survey, 2010–2013.

[1] Significantly different from non-Hispanic black and Hispanic men in the same age group. 2Significantly different from men aged 45 and over in the same race and ethnicity group.

Figure 4. Men who took medication or talked to a mental health professional, among men aged 18 and over who felt anxious or depressed every day, by age and race and ethnicity: United States, 2010–2013.

In fact, among insured men aged 18–44 with daily feelings of anxiety or depression, no statistical difference was observed between the racial and ethnic groups in the use of mental health treatments.

In contrast, racial and ethnic disparities in use of mental health treatments were observed regardless of family income. Among men aged 18–44 who felt anxious and depressed every day, non-Hispanic white men were 1.7 to 2.0 times as likely as non-Hispanic black and Hispanic men to have taken medication or talked to a mental health professional.

SUMMARY

Non-Hispanic black and Hispanic men were less likely than non-Hispanic white men to report having daily feelings of anxiety or depression, and this disparity was due to significant differences among younger men aged 18–44.

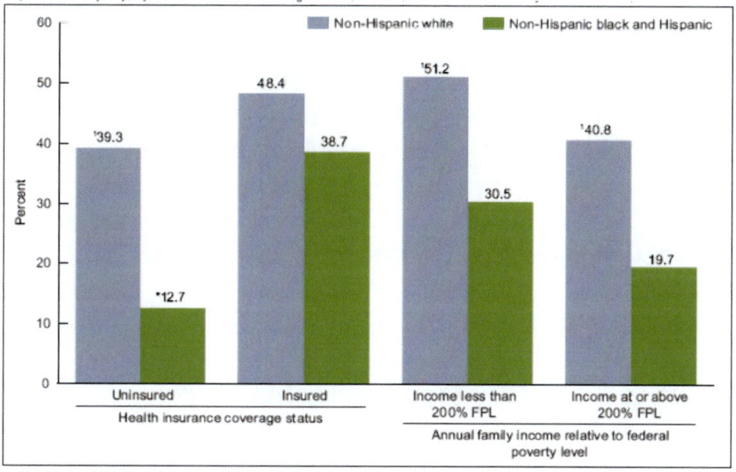

Source: CDC/NCHS, National Health Interview Survey, 2010–2013.
Note: FPL is federal poverty level.
[1] Figure 5does not meet standards of reliability or precision; estimate has a relative standard error of 35% (95% confidence interval: 6.2%–24.3%). 1Significantly different from non-Hispanic black and Hispanic men.

Figure 5. Men who took medication or talked to a mental health professional, among men aged 18–44 who felt anxious or depressed every day, by health insurance coverage status, income, and race and ethnicity: United States, 2010–2013.

This finding may seem to contradict other research revealing that rates of serious psychological distress [6] and depressive symptoms [7] are higher among Hispanic and non-Hispanic black persons than among non-Hispanic white persons. However, the findings in this report are based on a different measure of mental health symptoms (reported daily feelings) that considers frequency but not intensity of feelings. The findings in this report are also based on a different population (men only).

Younger men of color who reported daily feelings of anxiety or depression were less likely than their non-Hispanic white peers to take medication or talk to a mental health professional. This difference in treatment use was not observed for older men. Among the younger men, the racial and ethnic difference in treatment use was observed regardless of income.

Racial and ethnic differences in men's mental health treatment use appear to be driven by differences among younger uninsured men. The survey data cannot be used to determine if young men of color without health insurance, relative to young uninsured non-Hispanic white men, perceive less need for treatment, are less motivated to seek treatment, experience additional non-cost barriers when attempting to access mental health treatments, or more quickly stop using treatments that do not seem to be working. In focus groups, young men of color were particularly likely to say that mental illness and treatment seeking are signs of weakness and can bring shame and embarrassment to one's self and family [8]. Yet having health insurance coverage appeared to reduce the impact of such barriers; the observed racial and ethnic difference in treatment use was significantly smaller for younger insured men. Recent expansions of health insurance coverage may consequently reduce these racial and ethnic disparities.

DEFINITIONS

Daily feelings of anxiety or depression: Based on responses to the survey questions, "How often do you feel worried, nervous, or anxious?" and "How often do you feel depressed?" Answer choices were daily, weekly, monthly, a few times a year, or never.

Mental health treatments: Based on responses to the survey questions, "Do you take medication for these feelings?" and "During the past 12 months, have you seen or talked to any of the following health care providers about your own health ... A mental health professional such as a psychiatrist, psychologist, psychiatric nurse, or clinical social worker?"

Family income relative to federal poverty level: Based on family income, family size, and age using the U.S. Census Bureau's poverty thresholds for the previous calendar year. Imputed income files were used when income was missing.

Health insurance coverage status: Insured men include those who, at the time of interview, had any private health insurance, Medicare, Medicaid, Children's Health Insurance Program, a state-sponsored or other government-sponsored health plan, or a military plan. Men were defined as uninsured if they did not have any of these coverage types, had only Indian Health Service coverage, or had only a private plan that paid for one type of service, such as accidents or dental care.

Race and ethnicity: Ethnicity refers to Hispanic or Latino origin, and persons of Hispanic or Latino origin may be of any race. For conciseness, this report used shorter versions of the 1997 Office of Management and Budget terms for Hispanic or Latino origin and race. For example, the category "not Hispanic or Latino, white, single race" is referred to as "non-Hispanic white."

DATA SOURCE AND METHODS

The National Health Interview Survey (NHIS) is a multipurpose cross-sectional health survey that is fielded continuously by the Centers for Disease Control and Prevention's (CDC) National Center for Health Statistics. Interviews are conducted in respondent's homes, with telephone follow-up permitted if necessary. Analyses in this report were based on mental health and medication use data collected from a combined sample of 21,058 men aged 18 and over as part of the 2010 Quality of Life (QOL) and the 2011, 2012, and 2013 Adult Functioning and Disability (AFD) supplements to NHIS. Demographic and other health information (including contact with mental health professionals) were collected in the Household, Sample Adult Core, and Family Core components of NHIS. The QOL and AFD supplements were administered for a random subsample of NHIS sample adult respondents. For more information about NHIS, visit its website at: http://www.cdc.gov/nchs/nhis.htm.

Sampling weights were used to produce national estimates that are representative of the civilian noninstitutionalized U.S. population aged 18 and over [9]. Point estimates and statistical tests were calculated using SUDAAN software version 11.0 (RTI International, Research Triangle Park, N.C.) to account for the complex sample design of NHIS. Calculations excluded persons with unknown information. Sensitivity analyses were conducted to examine if the observed disparities with non-Hispanic white men differed for non-Hispanic black men relative to Hispanic men. No significant differences were observed, so estimates for non-Hispanic white men were compared with pooled estimates for non-Hispanic black and Hispanic men. Estimates reported for all men ("all races and ethnicities") include men with races and ethnicities other than non-Hispanic white, non-Hispanic black, and Hispanic. All comparisons were evaluated for statistical significance at the 0.05 level using two-sided tests.

Analyses of treatment use did not include the 4.6% of men who took medication for anxiety or depression but did not experience these feelings daily, perhaps as a result. The prevalence of medication use in the absence of daily feelings was lower for men of color (2.7%) relative to non-Hispanic white men (5.6%), and this difference did not vary by age or health insurance coverage status. Therefore, if the analyses in this report had included these men, treatment rates generally would have been higher, but all observed racial and ethnic differences would still be significant and the conclusions would not have changed.

About the Authors

Stephen J. Blumberg, Tainya C. Clarke, and Debra L. Blackwell are with CDC's National Center for Health Statistics, Division of Health Interview Statistics.

References

[1] Alegría M, Chatterji P, Wells K, Cao Z, Chen CN, Takeuchi D, et al. Disparity in depression treatment among racial and ethnic minority populations in the United States. *Psychiatr. Serv.* 59(11): 1264–72. 2008.

[2] Broman CL. Race differences in the receipt of mental health services among young adults. *Psychol. Serv.* 9(1): 38–48. 2012.

[3] HHS. Mental health: Culture, race, and ethnicity—A supplement to mental health: A report of the Surgeon General. Washington, DC. 2001.

[4] HHS. Mental health: A report of the Surgeon General. Washington, DC. 1999.

[5] Kessler RC, Berglund P, Demler O, Jin R, Merikangas KR, Walters EE. Lifetime prevalence and age-of-onset distributions of DSM-IV disorders in the National Comorbidity Survey Replication. *Arch. Gen. Psychiatry.* 62(6): 593–602. 2005.

[6] Weissman J, Pratt LA, Miller EA, Parker JD. Serious psychological distress among adults: United States, 2009–2013. NCHS data brief, no 203. Hyattsville, MD: National Center for Health Statistics. 2015.

[7] Pratt LA, Brody DJ. Depression in the U.S. household population, 2009–2012. NCHS data brief, no 172. Hyattsville, MD: National Center for Health Statistics. 2014.

[8] Thompson VLS, Bazile A, Akbar M. African Americans' perceptions of psychotherapy and psychotherapists. *Professional psychology: Research and practice* 35(1): 19–26. 2004.

[9] Parsons VL, Moriarity C, Jonas K, et al. Design and estimation for the National Health Interview Survey, 2006–2015. National Center for Health Statistics. Vital Health Stat 2(165). 2014.

In: Significant Health Statistics
Editor: Christopher Barrett
ISBN: 978-1-63484-563-2

Chapter 12

LEADING CAUSES OF DEATH CONTRIBUTING TO DECREASE IN LIFE EXPECTANCY GAP BETWEEN BLACK AND WHITE POPULATIONS: UNITED STATES, 1999–2013*

Kenneth D. Kochanek, MA, Elizabeth Arias, PhD, and Robert N. Anderson, PhD

KEY FINDINGS

Data from the National Vital Statistics System, Mortality

- The gap in life expectancy between the black and white populations decreased 2.3 years between 1999 and 2013 (5.9 to 3.6 years).
- The decrease in the gap was due to larger decreases in death rates for the black population for heart disease, cancer, and HIV disease.
- The gap in life expectancy between black and white males decreased 2.4 years between 1999 and 2013 (6.8 to 4.4 years).

---

* This is an edited, reformatted and augmented version of NCHS Data Brief, No. 218, issued by the National Center for Health Statistics, November 2015.

- The decrease in the gap was due to larger decreases in death rates for black males for HIV disease, cancer, and unintentional injuries.
- The gap in life expectancy between black and white females decreased 2.2 years between 1999 and 2013 (5.2 to 3.0 years).
- The decrease in the gap was due to larger decreases in death rates for black females for heart disease, HIV disease, and cancer.

The trend in U.S. life expectancy since 1900 has been one of gradual improvement [1]. Nevertheless, differences in life expectancy by race have persisted at least since official estimates were recorded. Measuring health disparities, including those in life expectancy, is part of the Healthy People 2020 recommendations [2]. In 1999, the difference in life expectancy between the white and black populations was 5.9 years. The gap decreased to 3.6 years in 2013. Black and white population differences in causes of death are explored to determine how they contribute to the decrease in the gap in life expectancy from 1999 through 2013.

Keywords: mortality, disparities, National Vital Statistics System

WHAT ARE THE RECENT TRENDS IN LIFE EXPECTANCY?

Life expectancy at birth increased steadily from 77.3 years in 1999 to 79.1 years in 2013 for the white population (2.3% increase) (Figure 1). For white males, the increase was from 74.6 years to 76.7 years (2.8% increase), and for white females, from 79.9 years to 81.4 years (1.9% increase).

Life expectancy at birth for the black population increased steadily from 71.4 years in 1999 to 75.5 years in 2013 (5.7% increase). For black males, the increase was from 67.8 years to 72.3 years (6.6% increase), and for black females, from 74.7 years to 78.4 years (5.0% increase).

HOW DID THE RACIAL GAP IN LIFE EXPECTANCY CHANGE OVER TIME?

In 2013, the difference in life expectancy at birth between the black and white populations was 3.6 years (Figure 2).

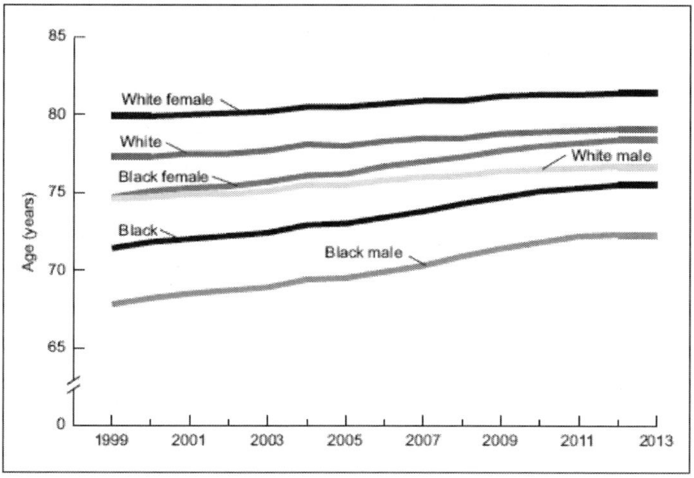

Source: CDC/NCHS, National Vital Statistics System, Mortality.

Figure 1. Life expectancy, by race and sex: United States, 1999–2013.

For black and white males, this difference was 4.4 years, and for black and white females, the difference was 3.0 years.

In 1999, the difference in life expectancy between the black and white populations was 5.9 years. For black and white males, this difference was 6.8 years, and for black and white females the difference was 5.2 years [1].

Between 1999 and 2013, the gap in life expectancy between the black and white populations decreased by 2.3 years. For black and white males, the decrease in the gap was 2.4 years, and for black and white females, the decrease in the gap was 2.3 years.

What Leading Causes of Death Influenced the Decrease in the Life Expectancy Gap Between the Black and White Populations from 1999 to 2013?

- The decrease in the gap in life expectancy between the black and white populations was due to larger decreases in death rates for the black population for heart disease, cancer, HIV disease, unintentional injuries, and perinatal conditions (Figure 3), which together accounted for 59.1% of the 2.3-year decrease in the gap.

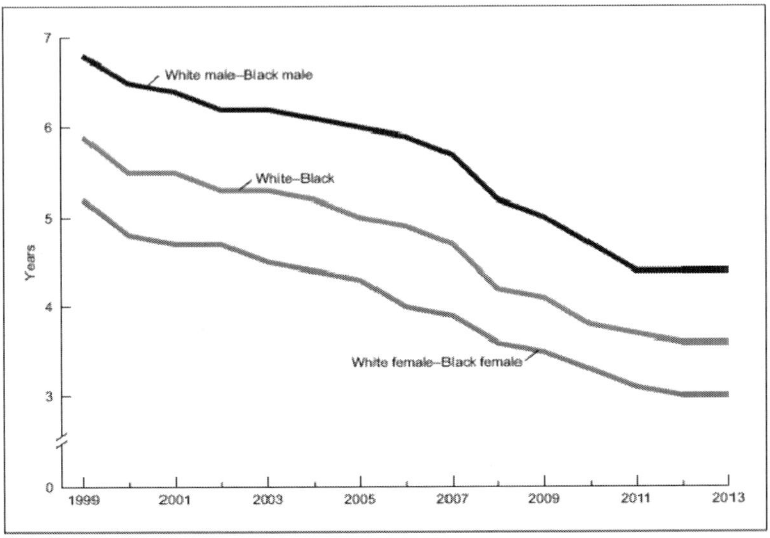

Source: CDC/NCHS, National Vital Statistics System, Mortality.

Figure 2. Differences in life expectancy between white and black populations, by sex: United States, 1999–2013.

- Greater decreases in heart disease mortality for the black population accounted for 0.370 year of the decrease in the gap in life expectancy.
- The decline in the gap was attenuated somewhat by greater increases in death rates from aortic aneurysm, Alzheimer's disease, and maternal conditions (Figure 3) for the black population. The increase in death rates for these causes accounted for 90.6% of the total increase in the gap.

What Leading Causes of Death Influenced the Decrease in the Gap in Life Expectancy Between the Black and White Male Populations from 1999 to 2013?

- Greater decreases in death rates for black males due to HIV disease, cancer, unintentional injuries, heart disease, and perinatal conditions (Figure 4) together accounted for 64.8% of the 2.4-year decrease in the gap.

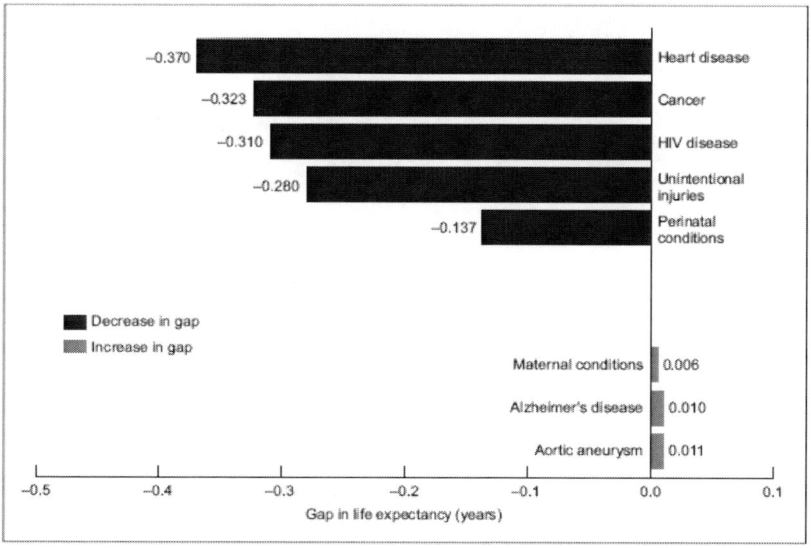

Source: CDC/NCHS, National Vital Statistics System, Mortality.

Figure 3. Contribution of leading causes of death to decrease in life expectancy gap between black and white populations: United States, 1999–2013.

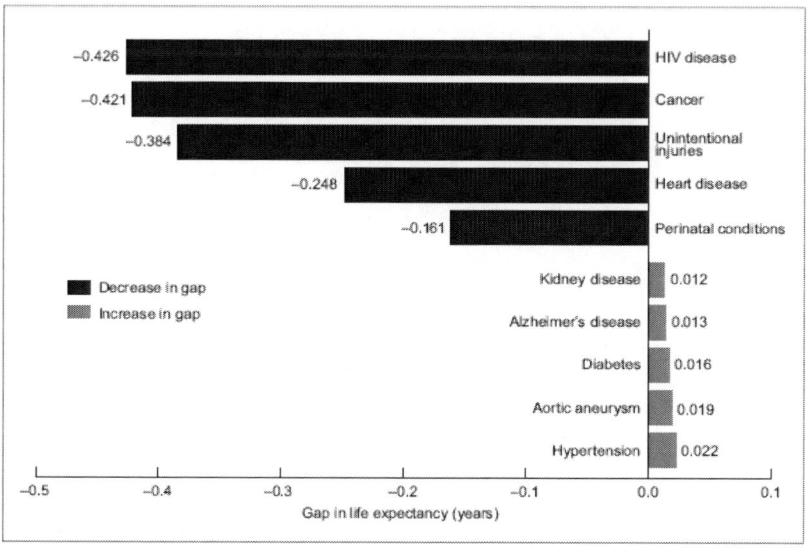

Source: CDC/NCHS, National Vital Statistics System, Mortality.

Figure 4. Contribution of leading causes of death to decrease in life expectancy gap between black and white males: United States, 1999–2013.

- Greater decreases in HIV disease mortality alone accounted for 0.426 year in the decrease in the gap in life expectancy between black and white males.
- Greater increases in death rates for black males due to hypertension, aortic aneurysm, diabetes, Alzheimer's disease, and kidney disease attenuated the decline in the gap between black and white males over the period.

What Leading Causes of Death Influenced the Decrease in the Gap in Life Expectancy Between the Black and White Female Populations from 1999 to 2013?

- Greater decreases in death rates for black females due to heart disease, HIV disease, cancer, diabetes, and unintentional injuries (Figure 5) together accounted for 54.7% of the 2.2-year decrease in the gap.
- Greater decreases in heart disease mortality alone accounted for 0.534 year in the decrease in the gap in life expectancy between black and white females.
- Greater increases in death rates for black females due to Alzheimer's disease, maternal conditions, and atherosclerosis attenuated the decline in the gap between black and white females over the same period.

Summary

Life expectancy at birth has increased steadily since 1900 to a record 78.8 years in 2013. But differences in life expectancy between the white and black populations still exist, despite a decrease in the life expectancy gap from 5.9 years in 1999 to 3.6 years in 2013. Differences in the change over time in the leading causes of death for the black and white populations have contributed to this decrease in the gap in life expectancy.

Between 1999 and 2013, the decrease in the life expectancy gap between the black and white populations was mostly due to greater decreases in mortality from heart disease, cancer, HIV disease, unintentional injuries, and perinatal conditions among the black population. Similarly, the decrease in the gap between black and white male life expectancy was due to greater decreases in death rates for HIV disease, cancer, unintentional injuries, heart disease, and perinatal conditions in black males. For black females, greater decreases in diabetes death rates, combined with decreased rates for heart disease and HIV disease, were the major causes contributing to the decrease in the life expectancy gap with white females.

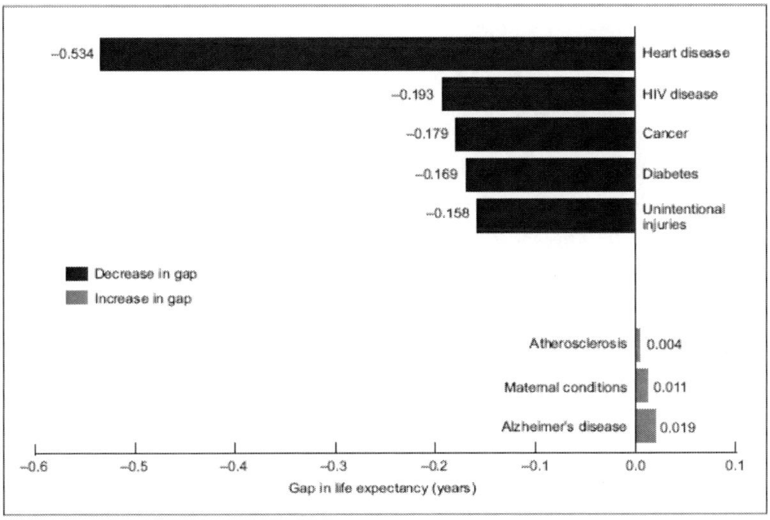

Source: CDC/NCHS, National Vital Statistics System, Mortality.

Figure 5. Contribution of leading causes of death to decrease in life expectancy gap between black and white females: United States, 1999–2013.

The decrease in the gap in life expectancy between the white and black populations would have been larger than 3.6 years if not for increases in death rates for the black population for aortic aneurysm, Alzheimer's disease, and maternal conditions. For black males, the causes that showed increases in death rates over white males were hypertension, aortic aneurysm, diabetes, Alzheimer's disease, and kidney disease, while the causes that showed increases in death rates for black females were Alzheimer's disease, maternal conditions, and atherosclerosis.

This *NCHS Data Brief* is the second in a series of data briefs that explore the causes of death contributing to differences in life expectancy between detailed ethnic and racial populations in the United States. The first data brief focused on the racial differences in life expectancy for a single year, 2010 [3].

DATA SOURCE AND METHODS

All data are from the 1999 and 2013 mortality files of the National Vital Statistics System. Life table methodology is explained in the NCHS reports "Deaths: Final Data for 2013" [1] and "United States Life Tables, 2010" [4]. A complete description of the Arriaga life table partitioning methodology is available elsewhere [5, 6].

DEFINITIONS

Cause-of-death classification: Medical information—including injury diagnoses and external causes of injury—that is entered on death certificates filed in the United States and classified and coded in accordance with the *International Statistical Classification of Diseases and Related Health Problems, Tenth Revision* (ICD–10) [7]. Corresponding cause-of-death categories and ICD–10 codes presented in this report are:

- Heart disease (Diseases of heart, I00–I09, I11, I13, I20–I51)
- Cancer (Malignant neoplasms, C00–C97)
- Unintentional injuries (Accidents, V01–X59, Y85–Y86)
- Alzheimer's disease (G30)
- Diabetes (Diabetes mellitus, E10–E14)
- Kidney disease (Nephritis, nephrotic syndrome and nephrosis, N00–N07, N17–N19, N25– N27)
- Hypertension (Essential hypertension and hypertensive renal disease, I10, I12, I15)
- Perinatal conditions (Certain conditions originating in the perinatal period, P00–P96)
- Aortic aneurysm (Aortic aneurysm and dissection, I71)
- HIV disease (Human immunodeficiency virus [HIV] disease, B20–B24)
- Maternal conditions (Pregnancy, childbirth and the puerperium, O00–O99)
- Atherosclerosis (I70)

Life expectancy: The average number of years that a group of infants would live if the group was to experience throughout life the age-specific death rates present in the year of birth. Also referred to as period, or current life expectancy [1].

About the Authors

Kenneth D. Kochanek, Elizabeth Arias, and Robert N. Anderson are with CDC's National Center for Health Statistics, Division of Vital Statistics, Mortality Statistics Branch.

References

[1] Xu JQ, Murphy SL, Kochanek KD. Deaths: Final data for 2013. National vital statistics reports; vol 64 no 2. Hyattsville, MD: National Center for Health Statistics. 2016 [Forthcoming].

[2] U.S. Department of Health and Human Services. Developing Healthy People 2020, Phase I report: Recommendations for the framework and format of Healthy People 2020, Appendix 11: Measuring health disparities and health equity. 2008. Available from: http://www.healthypeople.gov/2010/hp2020/advisory/PhaseI/appendix11.htm.

[3] Kochanek KD, Arias E, Anderson RN. How did cause of death contribute to racial differences in life expectancy in the United States in 2010? NCHS data brief, no 125. Hyattsville, MD: National Center for Health Statistics. 2013.

[4] Arias E. United States life tables, 2010. National vital statistics reports; vol 63 no 7. Hyattsville, MD: National Center for Health Statistics. 2014.

[5] Arriaga E. Measuring and explaining the change in life expectancies. Demography 21(1):83– 96. 1984.

[6] Arriaga EE. Changing trends in mortality decline during the last decades. In: Ruzicka L, Wunsch G, Kane P, editors. Differential mortality: Methodological issues and biosocial factors. Oxford, England: Clarendon Press. 1989.

[7] WHO. International statistical classification of diseases and related health problems, tenth revision (ICD–10). 2nd edition. Geneva, Switzerland. 2004.

INDEX

C

D

E

F

G

H

I

L

M

N

S

T

U

V

W

Y